Kevin Sharp
with Jeanne Gere

AVA RE NES-
ознакомление.

Tragedy's Gift
By Kevin Sharp with Jeanne Gere

Printed in Cincinnati, Ohio

ZassCo Publishing - www.zasscopublishing.com
for
Yada Yada Inc.
PO Box 967
Springhill, TN 37174

Editor: Sue Veldkamp
        www.matschca.com

Cover Design: Marc Giguere
              Sue Veldkamp

Photo Credits: Nancy Andrews

Library of Congress Control Number:
2004107793

ISBN: 0-9758512-1-7

Dedication

This book is dedicated to the memory of Carter T. "Coach" Williams. We love and miss you.

Index

Kevin Sharp Friends Club
P.O. Box 888
Camino, CA 95709
ksfanclb@innercite.com

Thanks for your support!
Marlene Urso, President
Elaine Mattei, Vice President

Introduction

When I was first asked to consider a new writing assignment with a country music artist, I was reluctant. The only thing I knew about Kevin Sharp was that he once had cancer and more recently, some number one hit songs. I concluded that he must have been having a pity party about his past and self-absorbed about his present success. The prospect was not very enticing to say the least. I didn't know if I was up for the task because I never did well when it came to people with large egos or fragile temperaments.

However, eighteen months and one extraordinary book later, I am pleased to stand corrected. I sit here writing these comments with a whole new attitude about Kevin Sharp. I have an overwhelming amount of respect for him as a person, an artist and a humanitarian.

From our very first meeting when Kevin recalled his childhood and the love he felt for his family, I was hooked. It was clear to me that I had misjudged him completely. I wholeheartedly wanted to help him write his story.

Then one day in the midst of working, Kevin told me that he didn't look forward to our sessions because they brought back too many painful memories and feelings from difficult times. That's when I knew we were working on a story that would really touch people's hearts. He was not going to compromise the truth to spare his own suffering. I watched Kevin wrestle with the past and go through torment all over again so his story could be told with honesty. He never held back the truth to spare feelings or to sugarcoat the severity of the situation.

I could see the compassion on his face as he talked about the sacrifice his family and so many other families made for their children. His longing to make a difference was evident every time his mind wandered back to his days in the pediatrics ward. His excitement for music can light up a room, and his desire to speak about hope and strength and never giving up is clearly a driving force in his life.

This book is just the tip of the iceberg for Kevin Sharp. He has so many more things to say and many more books in his heart. I know life is going to continue to take Kevin in many directions, but I also know that Kevin is well equipped to handle the good, bad, and anything in between. He walks hand in hand with faith, kindness, hope, love and perseverance.

I am proud to call Kevin Sharp my friend, and I am honored to be a part of this book.

With love and respect,

Jeanne Gere

Forward

"Pain, I know it well. I lived with it in Hell." These lyrics were sung by Kevin in the church musical "Joshua," when he played a Roman Centurion Officer dealing with pain because he'd been part of King Herod's rampage to kill babies at the time of Christ's birth. Kevin told us then that every song he sings must have meaning to him. The feelings he put into singing this song came from his soul because he understands mental, physical and emotional pain.

Our son has told us that he wishes he could make a difference in people's lives, to touch people and make their days better. He has no idea how many lives he has touched and the difference he has made. His "Friends Club" staff has, on many occasions, sent us copies of letters that prove this to be true.

One letter came from a mother who said she heard Kevin singing, "Nobody

Knows" over the loud speaker while shopping at Wal-Mart. She could not leave the store until she purchased the CD because "Nobody Knows" said it all. She mentioned her young son could determine her mood by the song she was listening to. If it was "Nobody Knows," then he knew she was feeling blue, but when it was "Strength to Love," he knew her spirits were up. The letter said, "Thanks for your music." It was signed at the end with an address and phone number.

"I'm alright, I'm okay and I'll live to fight another day because I've got hope and that's enough until I find the strength to love."

A week or so after the first letter, a second one arrived stating that she had been sitting at the dining room table reading over her divorce papers when the telephone rang. Her son answered it and started shouting as he ran toward her. "It's Kevin Sharp, Mom." This experience is something our son never told us about. He's like that. He doesn't like to boast; he helps when he can and it goes way beyond cancer-related incidents.

We appreciate the Make-A-Wish Foundation. Kevin wasn't our first experience with them. Our granddaughter Danielle was 4 ½ years old when she was diagnosed with Rhabdomyosarcoma. Make-A-Wish sent the family to Disneyland in California as her wish. So when Kevin was diagnosed, his sister Lisa suggested contacting Make-A-Wish again. Kevin was scared and angry. The wish made a difference. It gave him a reason to live and we are eternally grateful. We have, since then, worked continually as wish granters and fund raisers for the Foundation.

We have personally visited with families with sick children and listened to their dreams. We have been able to be part of their fulfillment of trips to Disney World, new computers, wide screen televisions, shopping sprees and a horse like Trigger, as well as meeting Dale Evans and others. As we look into the eyes of new Make-A-Wish families, we know they don't realize what lies ahead and how much strength will be needed. The whole family fights for survival.

As Kevin's mother, I had the privilege of going to the Make-A-Wish National Conference in Phoenix to accept in his place a "Wish Grantor of the Year" award because Kevin was in the hospital having surgery to repair his damaged hip. We realized then he had learned that by giving back he was gaining strength. Make-A-Wish gave to him and he was giving back.

Nothing thrills us more than to see Kevin perform on stage and now that he is an inspirational speaker, it thrills us even more. At every concert he says that we should learn to accept the differences in each other and love one another more. We are proud of our son and this book. It's another way for him to reach out. If he can help one other person, he feels he has accomplished a great deal.

We are proud parents of all of our children, grandchildren and great-grandchildren.

Blessings All,

Glen and Elaine Sharp

Preface

Maybe this was Heaven and I really did die, and now I get to realize my wildest dreams. Imagine, me sitting in a seat directly behind Garth Books, nominated for, "New Male Vocalist of the Year." Imagine, me on an awards show I had watched time and time again on TV in my living room.

I had so many mixed emotions that night. The excitement of being somewhere I had fantasized about my entire life, sitting among my heroes who were now considered my peers. Let's face it; it's not every day that someone like me has moments like these.

I was sitting next to my dad, watching him enjoy this adventure as much, if not more than I was. I cringed as I watched him tap Garth on the shoulder numerous times to ask questions. I felt embarrassed like in those crazy nightmares where I had just walked into school and forgot my pants!

But the thrill lessened any feelings other than unbelievable.

Then it hit me, this couldn't be Heaven because I also felt sadness welled up inside me as I remembered the loss of my dear friend and an important part of my management team, Jeff Yoke, who died in a car crash just two days earlier while picking up my tuxedo for this glamorous event. His efforts were a part of the reason I was able to be in this place.

All of these emotions bubbling around inside of me must be the reason for the tears streaming down my face. Joy with sadness, pleasure with pain; I was no stranger to these ironies. Up to this point, my life was full of them.

Growing Up

Most of my early childhood memories are a blur. I grew up in a home with my parents and a large family of eight children. I was born on December 10, 1970. My dad, Glen Sharp, was a bishop in our church, which would equate to a priest or pastor in other denominations. Dad owned a legal company that provided multiple services to lawyers and the court system. He juggled church and work with the grace of a gazelle. The importance of attending church was greatly instilled in us during my upbringing.

My father also loved music. I know he dreamed of being a singer in his younger years. If he hadn't met my mom when he did, I think he might have tried for a career as a performer. In my eyes he was a successful performer. In fact, I thought he was the best. I know that my mom and the rest of us were glad he turned his focus to his family.

Right before I was born, Dad made commercials for the car company he worked for. Rumor has it that his favorite sales pitch was that he, "had cars coming out of his ears," and in one commercial he actually wore little cars in his ears. I guess a true performer will do whatever it takes to entertain his audience. I am glad my peers were only newborns at that time!

Dad had my older siblings take instrument lessons; one playing the piano, one the drums, guitar, etc., and then he organized this, "Partridge Family" type group and they would play and sing at church functions. They did that for about two years until the older kids lost interest and refused to do it any more. After they revolted, I was old enough to do a solo act for my parents. I was always ready to belt out a tune whether I was asked to or not.

My mom, Elaine, was a schoolteacher who took early retirement before I was born so she could raise our family. I really have fond recollections of her being a stay-at-home mom. With eight children, I can't imagine how she did it, but she was very good at being a homemaker.

We lived in Cottonwood, California in a small home with three bedrooms and two bathrooms. If you do the math, the ratio of kids to rooms was slightly off by a room or two! We had bunk beds out on the back porch where my older brothers slept. We did what we had to do to make things work. We raised chickens, pigs, sheep, goats, a cow and a bull. I guess one could call it a small farm. That's what my dad liked about living in the country.

One event that sticks out in my mind the most about Cottonwood is that I used to keep a nightlight plugged in next to my bed and one night while I was asleep it shorted out and my hair caught on fire. To this day, my mother cannot explain why she woke up in the middle of the night to check on me, but as she did, she was able to put out the fire and keep me from being burned. The only explanation that makes sense to me involves guardian angels and God's favor in my life even at an early age.

A Dry Night

By the time I was six years old, I was what I would now consider to be a professional worrier. I worried about everything, as though it was my personal mission to dread, run scenarios in my mind, and sweat out every situation I could think of. If that wasn't bad enough, it was also the time I started to wet the bed.

In most cases, six would be the age when bed-wetting would start to wane. Not in my case. As if I needed something else to dread!

At the time, I was sharing a room with my brother Richard and my foster brother Jeremiah. I tried with everything I had to hide my "secret" from them as long as I could. The embarrassment and shame I felt was overwhelming. I would sneak my sheets into the garbage every morning and then when no one was around, I'd slip them into the laundry basket so my mother could wash them. I thought I could continue this method forever, but my tactic only worked for a while. The smell of urine is very distinct and it didn't take too many nights of "accidents" before my brothers started to catch on. This didn't help our relationship any. No one wanted to sleep with that smell in the room, and I can't say that I blamed them.

The embarrassment was worse when I had friends over and they would ask why my room smelled like pee. I learned quickly to make up stories to cover for my secret.

My worrying took on a new dimension. Before bed-wetting, I worried about things that didn't really concern me first hand, but now I had personal humiliation to contend with. I wondered who would find out.

What would I do if I had to attend a sleep over? What would my friends do if they knew? I thought I was going to die. I felt like a freak and an alien.

I was six years old when the first episode occurred and this problem continued for three years. The impact it had on me was overwhelming and the emotional damage stayed with me long after the wetting stopped.

As an adult, I can see that being a worrier in the first place had everything to do with my problem. I always felt different than everyone else. I never felt a sense of security and I had a distorted sense of expectations that I thought were being placed on me.

I can't remember being told that it was okay to have accidents or weaknesses. I was never aware that other people went through similar situations or had to overcome the same obstacle as I did. I felt like an outsider, different, weird. I look back and wish that I could undo some of that anxiety. I wish someone had been looking for the signs of stress that accompany a child reaching the breaking point. I didn't have an adult in my life that was gauging my stress levels.

In reality, I was probably no different than most other kids in my school. The only problem was that I didn't know it. No one ever told me that I was, "normal." I didn't have anyone to share my fears with. I never felt free to be emotionally transparent with my family or friends. The pressure to be "like everyone else" and to quietly blend in was the focal point of my existence. My self-consciousness was self-inflicted.

On The Move

My parents were always ready to lend a helping hand. There were constantly new faces at the dinner table, or foster brothers and sisters weaving in and out of our lives. I had a foster brother from the Indian Exchange Program who lived with us for seven years. Helping others has been, and to this day is a determination of my father's. He never misses an opportunity to be in the service of another.

In 1974 we moved to Sacramento. Once again, our new house was small in comparison to the size of the family. Thankfully we only stayed there a short time until we moved to Fair Oaks, just outside of Sacramento. That home was much larger and made things more comfortable for everyone. No matter where we lived, my mother always made a nice environment for us and we never felt poor or needy, even when finances were tight.

Certain things were important to my mother. She wanted us to have dinner together as a family. We always went to church on Sunday, but most of all, even from the earliest age, she wanted us to be conscientious and to choose to do the right thing. Looking back on that now, I am sure that my sense of responsibility and challenge to be an upright person was developed during that stage in my life.

After dinner on Saturday nights was an event for us. When I was still pre-school age, my mom would draw a bath and one at a time she would take the five younger ones into the tub, wash us down, and then wrap us in a towel. It was only after I was a little older that I realized the importance of being close to first in the line up, as she would use the same water for all of us! I don't know if I recall that experience with fondness or not!

There was a great amount of fun to be had whenever it rained, because the backfields would flood with water and we would go out there and catch frogs. There were literally hundreds of frogs and my brothers and I found every imaginable way to play with them. Unfortunately for the frogs, we owned a bee-bee gun. My father and brother Larry, who had a deep love for animals, soon helped us to understand that our idea of fun was not the same as the frogs. We didn't use the bee-bee gun to play with frogs after that.

Things were so simple and innocent at that time. We had chores to do every day, and the reward for doing them was our Saturday allowance. My mother would give us our money and one of the older kids would walk the little ones to the Circle K Convenience Store to buy whatever candy we wanted. My little sister and I looked forward to that trip every week. It gave us a feeling of independence and reward for a job well done. Fifty cents went a long way back then and it seemed as though we bought a lot of candy for our money.

My father was a hard-working man. His business quickly became very successful, making it necessary for my mom to jump in and help. They both worked very long hours every day. I think their dedication to business and the family was where I got my belief that as long as I lived a good and moral life, nothing bad would ever happen to me. I watched them strive to be good people and wanted to emulate those qualities in my own life.

I took piano lessons until I was eight, but never really mastered playing it. I didn't mind because I never did have the discipline it required to become proficient at playing an instrument as I found out with the trumpet and many other instruments I picked up over the years. Besides, just because my brother Greg had mastered the trumpet didn't mean I could (as the band teacher soon found out.) I liked singing better because it came more naturally to me. From the time I was very small, about 4 or 5, I would put on musical shows for my family. I would make tickets to sell (but mostly I had to give them away for free,) and I would stand on the coffee table in the living room and sing or lip sync to Barry Manilow, Glen Campbell or John Denver songs.

I eventually branched out into the neighborhood. I would deliver singing telegrams to my neighbors whether they wanted one or not. One time I got a one-dollar tip and dreamed of making it big as a singer! I consider that to be my first road tour!

In 1979, my dad's company caused him to put in so many hours that it nearly drove him to his grave with worry. His health began to fail. On his doctor's advice, he sold his company, we packed up again, and this time moved from sunny California to Weiser, Idaho.

This was the first time I had ever experienced a sense of loss. I had to leave my best friend and neighbor behind. He was someone that I spent a part of every day with, and now we were separated. I couldn't imagine not seeing him again. I can remember crying for the better part of five hours into the trip.

My two older sisters Lisa and Mary decided to stay behind and finish their schooling in California. This also crushed me because Lisa had always been very good to me and Mary was the hero of my life. She was athletic and excelled at every sport. I wanted to be around her every minute and she never seemed to mind. She always let me tag along despite the ten-year age difference. She never made me feel like a pesky kid brother. I loved her so much that being separated from her nearly broke my heart. Still, to this day I have never forgotten at an early age, while in Cub Scouts, what Lisa had done for me. I had just come in last place for the third year in a row in the Cub Scout Derby. (My dad and I were never very good at the car-building phase.)

Some of the other fathers and sons used space technology to assure a win.

Needless to say I was very embarrassed, again. So, without thinking and with tears running down my face, I threw my car into the street. Later that night I was upset because I now wanted my car. It was Lisa who drove me around looking for it. When we finally found it, it had been smashed by passing cars, but never the less, I was happy to have my little wooden car back. What my sister did for her little brother will always be a special memory in my heart

Leaving them behind was an emotionally challenging time for me. It didn't feel as though anyone understood my pain.

We moved to Weiser, Idaho, where my dad bought a local restaurant. I think his plan was to relieve his stress by owning a quiet little diner in a small rural area. Believe me when I tell you he couldn't have picked a smaller town. Weiser had about four thousand people and no convenience stores and not even a McDonalds! It was the epitome of a one-horse town. I couldn't imagine what I would do for fun, or how we planned on living there for any length of time. One saving grace was that at 14 I could get a driver's license. Only six years to go! It was Weiser that my family would call home for the next 8 years.

As part of the real estate agreement, our new house was the one next door to the restaurant. Although it made the most financial sense, my father still had to put up with his six kids' constant complaints about it being too small. Dad's plan was to find a bigger house as soon as possible, but doing so took a lot longer than anticipated. This caused many arguments between my parents and us kids. To this day we joke about the house being so cold that icicles formed on the *inside* of the windows. The first winter in Idaho was brutal for this California boy.

Once I settled into school I quickly found friends, and things were good for the next several years. The kids in town thought we were rich because we owned a restaurant. Although we were far from rich, my dad treated my friends to free ice cream, which I thought was very cool of him to do! We raised a few farm animals, I mowed lawns to make spending money, and the restaurant was doing well, although it wasn't much less stress for my father. Dad seemed to wrestle with his decision to move to Idaho, wondering if it was the right one for the family. I think he found solace knowing that a small town upbringing would be good for us and in hindsight he definitely made the right decision.

When I entered the fifth grade I started playing Little League Football. I played for the Broncos and I was proud. Our team went to the championships that year. I remember that season better than any of the others for two reasons. First, we shared the championship with the Weiser

Cowboys. It was the only football championship I ever shared with a team in my entire school football career. We were down by six points and I was the one who scored the touchdown that tied the game, and secondly, because in that same season, I was hit so hard that I got the breath knocked out of me, which caused me to swallow my tongue. I went into convulsions and had to be rushed off the field. At nine years old the excitement of winning definitely outweighed my fear of suffocation. However, the fear was always with me in the back of my mind and remained there until I was out of high school.

Many things were starting to change. Lisa and Ron were getting married and Mary was off at college on a basketball scholarship. It felt like life was spinning out of control, or at least out of *my* control. The town's police department felt differently about Ron growing and maturing since he was known to get speeding tickets quite regularly. There was even a cartoon in the local paper starring Ron and the sheriff making light of their many run-ins.

By the time I was thirteen years old, family rules and traditions started to get a little more lenient than they had been before. It was no big deal if I ate dinner in front of the TV. Partly because my mom didn't have time to make an elaborate dinner and partly because I was seventh in a line up of eight children and my parents seemed to relax a little. There wasn't anything new that I could do or say that one of my siblings hadn't expressed or experienced before me. We always had an ongoing debate about who had it tougher, the younger or the older kids. I think as my mom raised more and more kids, she just didn't panic about things any more. So my being younger I had less structure, but the older kids enjoyed my parents' excitement of first experiences. The trade off seemed even to me. All in all, each of us had a happy childhood.

By the time I reached eight or nine, my parents had already instilled a strong foundation of family unity and acceptable behavior, so I knew right from wrong. I can't remember causing them any major grief. I could be recalling it all wrong, but I don't think I am.

I played sports throughout junior high with the exception of eighth grade. I injured my leg and it bothered me for the entire season. I think I worried about something being very wrong with my leg at that time, but I never wanted to bother my parents with my suspicions.

Because I was a natural worrier as a child, every time I had a report due in school, I would get absolutely sick with anxiety. Then, after I handed it in and received a good grade, I promised myself I would never agonize like that again. But, sure enough, the very next time, I was sick with worry all over again. I was never able to break that pattern throughout my school age years.

As I got older, I found more things to concern myself with. For example, I would fear my friends seeing me shop at K-Mart for clothes or Payless for shoes. I didn't think anyone else's family had to worry about money or being "thrifty." I was constantly thinking about what I would wear to school and if someone would notice that I had worn the same blue jeans twice in one week. To compound the issue, I also thought I was the only kid on the planet that worried about what other kids would think of me. It never crossed my mind that everyone was insecure and feared peer criticism. I prayed that no one would think I was poor.

I sometimes worried about situations that didn't even have anything to do with me. There were nights when I would lay awake and just fret over all I heard or saw on the news that day or discussions my parents would have about finances, or about experiences my brothers or sisters were

going through.   I couldn't seem to just relax and enjoy being a kid.

Another time in particular that caused me tremendous worry was my fiddle playing days. When we settled into Weiser, my mother thought fiddle lessons would encourage my love for music. Weiser was the home of the National Fiddle Festival that was held the third week of every June. Each year the town's population would double as a result of the festival, so an obvious selection of instruments and lessons would be the fiddle. Mom bought me a new fiddle and I set out to get ready for the festival. I soon found out that I was not cut out for playing the fiddle any more than I was cut out for playing the piano. I still lacked the discipline and had no patience to play. I was a singer! I decided to quit. Then I proceeded to spend weeks worrying about the money I wasted. Finally, mom sold the fiddle and I could stop feeling guilty. She made her money back. The funny thing about that situation was that she never gave it a second thought. I was the only one losing any sleep over it.

I was very good at sports. I played football in high school and worked out with weights. A part of who I was revolved around a healthy lifestyle and a physically fit body. I found a great deal of comfort and identity in being a non-smoker & non-drinker. I worked hard at being a worthy teammate. I wanted so much to be like my older brothers Greg and Richard. They were big and strong and seemed to have the respect of their peers. Richard was so successful at wrestling that I wanted to be the same. I was so worried about what my brothers thought of me I got caught up trying to be who I thought I should be, instead of being happy with whom I wanted to be. I know they never realized just how much I wanted to impress them. Ultimately I just ended up trying too hard and looking like I just wanted their and everyone else's attention focused on me. I assure them now that wasn't my intention.

I also sang in the school choir and performed in churches with my family. Participating in both activities seemed like a slight contradiction for my friends and teachers, but I felt gifted in both areas and decided to be dedicated to both.

I had my first girlfriend when I was in eighth grade. My parents had a rule that we couldn't date until we were sixteen, so it was more of a school day romance. Natalie was my first love. She was my first kiss, and my days began and ended with thoughts of her. I could not imagine anything about my life changing.

My fourteenth year could not have been more perfect. I had sports, a driver's license, music, a girlfriend, and decent grades that kept me out of trouble and in the good graces of my parents. I loved my life, and to my surprise, Weiser, Idaho had become home to me.

It was the summer going into my sophomore year that my life was about to change one more time. The business that was so likely to kill my father back in California all of those years ago had once again reared its ugly head. The gentleman who had purchased it from dad had done a less than stellar job of managing things and stood to lose everything. Everything included the money he owed my father for the initial purchase.

Limited options had my father packing us up and going back to Sacramento once again. We actually moved back into the same house we left all those years before. My dad jumped head first into saving the failing company, and I was struggling with the devastation of leaving behind everything I loved, including Natalie.

I spent hours listening to our favorite songs, remembering all of the talks we had and the way she made me feel when we were together. I missed her so much I cried for hours knowing that I was helpless and couldn't change anything to bring us back together. The love I felt for

Natalie stayed fresh in my heart long after I left Weiser.

I started my sophomore year at Bella Vista High School. Everything was different than what I was used to. The culture shock was overwhelming. Drinking, partying, and mediocre grades were not considered the wrong things; they were now the cool things to do. Everything felt backward to me except for football. I made the team and began playing as soon as we returned to California. Football became my saving grace. It was my success on the field that made my new surroundings and adapting a little easier to handle. However, it took me months to stop feeling the pain of leaving Natalie behind.

It wasn't long after my dad took his business back that he suffered his first heart attack. What the doctors had predicted eight years before had come to pass as a result of stress and long hours at work. It was the first time I had ever realized that my parents wouldn't live forever. Dad needed help that surpassed what my mother could give, so we all pitched in and came to his aid. The timing worked well for me because I felt over-extended being on the school basketball team, and this was a way to bow out without hurting my teammates or ruining my relationship with the coach. I was glad to be helping my dad in any way I could. I spent my afternoons and evenings doing filing, organizing paperwork and anything else that would ease the stress for my parents. My brothers and sisters each had their part to do and did it without too much complaining or feeling put upon. It was really my mom and older siblings who stepped up and took on the heavy load in order to just keep us afloat. I was just beginning to see how strong of a woman my mother was and how she was the backbone of this family.

The Diagnosis

In the summer of 1987, I began having knee and back pain, which caused me to limp. After a visit to the doctor it was determined that I must have gotten a sports injury that was slow to heal. In my senior year I didn't feel well enough to play football or basketball; I lost a lot of my physical strength and at that point was having a difficult time with one particular coach. I couldn't understand why he wanted to work with kids. He didn't seem very good at it. I was feeling weaker by the day and I had to let my dreams and plans of playing college football go. Quitting the team turned out to be a lot harder than I'd thought it would be. It was really a difficult time for me.

My buddies and I used to have this little joke; I would sing songs as I bench pressed over 200 lbs. One day we were playing around and I dropped the set on my chest. I just laughed it off so no one would know how sick I was becoming. Many visits to the doctor still concluded that I was suffering from a prolonged injury.

I met a new girl, Kasey, the summer before my senior year. It was two years since I had last seen Natalie, and I had to let my heart move on. Although I had dated other girls, Kasey and I hit it off and remained an item all year. Our first date was to the mall to go clothes shopping for school. I thought she was the most beautiful girl in California. Kasey and her family quickly became like my own family and I had a bond with them that I felt would last a lifetime. We had a wonderful teenage romance.

During that time of my senior year I regularly suffered from uncontrollable sweats and had extremely dark circles under my eyes. When Kasey and I went to my senior prom I had to use crutches so I could make it through the entire night. I was having so much trouble standing for long periods of time during choir class that I asked to be excused from the last concert of the year. My director assumed I was having a bad attitude and warned me if I didn't show up for the concert I would fail the class. I nearly collapsed that night and still no one could provide any answers.

So many times my friends took offense because they couldn't understand why I chose to stay home on the weekend when they were all going out to have fun. It was hard to imagine that I could feel sick all the time or be in pain and never have an explanation for it. They took it as a sign that I would rather be alone, but nothing could have been further from the truth. I loved being a teenager and wanted to experience all the excitement life had to offer.

One day when we were hanging out, some of my buddies and I made a movie about my health dilemma. I took my friend's video camera and we did a spoof about me being in a hospital bed dying from a mysterious leg injury. I had tubes and IV's hanging from every part of my body. It was funny at the time because I was always telling my pals not to bump into me or to be careful of my leg if we were horsing around. This unexplained injury became a joke to us.

As my senior year progressed, so did my mystery ailment. It took all of the power I could muster up to limp my way through my graduation ceremony. I had been feeling sick and was in pain for almost three years and felt so helpless because not one doctor could find anything wrong with me. The outward physical signs of weakness and weight loss didn't seem to cause any curiosity to the medical world. I was frustrated and my family felt vulnerable.

After graduation, I heard about an audition for Music Circus, a summer stock group that allowed amateurs an opportunity to work with professional actors and singers who were between paying jobs. I desperately wanted to be a part of that show. They performed different shows every week. The first was going to be South Pacific. I hoped that my years of singing in the choir and at church with my family would be enough experience to get me through the auditions. I knew that if I got the chance, I had what it would take to be a performer.

I was sick the day of the open auditions with all the actors, dancers and singers together in a cattle call. I did, however, have the opportunity to do a private audition a few days later. I really wanted to be a part of this group because it would allow me to get closer to my dreams of being a singer, and would also be worth a few college credits through an extension program I enrolled in.

I was very nervous, which seemed to be to the delight of the director. One line into my song he stopped me to give direction.

The next time I got through two lines and he stopped me again. I never did finish the song. Feeling defeated, I went home to wait. I never expected to hear from those people again.

In a few days, I received a call informing me that I had gotten the part. That was exactly what I needed to put my illness and feelings of frailty behind me. I thought that this would be the beginning of a new and healthier me and that I would get this "performance bug" out of my system in enough time to go to college in the fall.

After days of rehearsals, I was struggling to keep up with the rest of the cast, but I was determined to make this work. The first Show was *South Pacific*, which required my character to have a military look. The director wanted me to cut my hair, which at that time was down the middle of my back. I told him that I didn't want to because I was going to be a singer and short hair was not my image.

He laughed and called me a, "nobody that doesn't have an image." I knew right then and there that I was in the professional arena. I cut my hair! The very next play was Oliver! I needed long hair for that role and ended up having to wear a wig. Who said showbiz was easy?

The effort to keep up the grueling show schedule proved difficult for me. We performed one show at night and rehearsed for the next show during the day. I was doing my best to hide my fatigue. The schedule was draining every ounce of energy I had. I was required to do a fight scene in *Seven Brides for Seven Brothers* with *Days of Our Lives* soap opera star Peter Reckell. I was very excited to be working with a television star. Everything was going so well, I was doing what I loved to do, I was gaining recognition for my work and I was happy. However, during rehearsals I just couldn't handle the physical strain and collapsed on stage! The director was very concerned for me, but his shows needed to go on. He had no choice but to let me go. Although he made sincere and genuine apologies, I was devastated. I felt alive on stage and letting go of this opportunity killed my spirit. I needed to find answers.

Kasey's parents were so concerned about my failing health that they insisted that I see an acupuncturist that they had visited. During one of my treatments, as the acupuncturist started to put the tiny needle into my left leg, it shot across the room and hit the wall. He ordered me to see my doctors and explain his findings to them. Still I received no diagnosis or help. It was just business as usual for the medical industry.

By this time, the physical pain was unbearable. I would lay awake without sleeping for days on end. My mother would spend hours sitting by me trying to comfort my weak body. I couldn't eat, sleep or think. I was consumed with sickness and pain. Every inch of my body and every corner of my mind were preoccupied with wondering what was wrong with me. I knew that an old sports injury could not cause this downhill spiral I was experiencing. Once again I went to the hospital seeking answers.

After another emergency room visit, I was given a prescription pain reliever to help me get some rest. We returned home in the middle of the night and my dad put me to bed.

The next morning Kasey came over to visit, and as she entered my room she found me there unable to breathe, hanging on to life by a thin thread. I was literally fighting for every lungful of air as though it would be my last. I was dying.

She screamed for my parents and the scene that ensued was one of the most terrifying memories of my life. I could hear the commotion, the yelling, the sirens getting louder as the paramedics drew closer to the house. I could feel the panic, but I was helpless. I saw neighbors gathering outside in the street as they wheeled me to the ambulance. I was given oxygen, and could hear the EMTs talking about my vital signs. This was the first time I ever saw fear in my father's face. I could see in his expression that something was seriously wrong. I knew that my fear was the worst I had ever felt. I sensed the life that I was barely holding on to fighting to leave my body. My fear was immeasurable. They were bringing me back to the same hospital I had visited just hours before.

When I reached the emergency room it was chaos. My parents were in a state of horror. Kasey and her mom got there before I did. Kasey was sure that I had died in my bedroom. She was inconsolable.

Although I had been to this same emergency room many times, most recently just hours before, everything was different now. I was being admitted for blood tests, X-rays, and an MRI. Finally, while I was at death's door, everything I was complaining about for three years was being taken seriously.

After being admitted, I was met by two doctors. They both had a startling fear on their faces. I knew that falling back on the sports injury diagnosis was no longer an option. I was not prepared for the discussions that came next.

That day I became an official adult. The doctors no longer wanted to explain things to my parents. My diagnosis was not going to be buffered by the smiles and hugs of my Mom and Dad. It was a straightforward discussion about a bone cancer called Ewing's Sarcoma, tumors, leg amputation and signing papers. I was now being probed and stuck with Intravenous needles and given unknown medications. There were no choices. My leg had a tumor. If I didn't agree to have it amputated I would surely die. I couldn't comprehend my situation. How could life get any worse? How could I escape this overwhelming panic that consumed me?

As the test results slowly trickled in, my diagnosis changed. I no longer just had cancer in my leg; they had also found a spot on one of my lungs. My oncologists looked directly into my eyes and told me that amputation was no longer an option. My odds of survival had dropped dramatically. My doctors' hope and positive attitudes seemed to disappear. They feared that there wasn't much they could do, but assured me that they would keep me comfortable in any event.

The cancer was too far along; there were no proven drugs to keep me alive. Once again as an adult, it was suggested that I spend my last few months of life at home with my family.

That day was chaotic. I remember people yelling in the hospital hallway. I could see my mother trying to hide her grief. My dad never left my side. This news was more than Kasey could bear. She was in shock. The faces of the people who entered my room spoke volumes. I felt horrible for them because there was nothing anyone could say. No words could make things better; no amount of tears could cry this monster away. I was living on borrowed time.

The next day, I don't know exactly how or why, but when the oncologist returned to my room, he asked if I wanted to try an experimental treatment. He had a thick stack of papers with him for me to read over before I needed to make a decision. I immediately flipped to the back page, asked for his pen and signed the release. Why read about possible side effects or life endangering episodes? I had no reason not to try. At that moment I knew the true meaning of the adage, "Nothing to lose."

Radiation and Chemotherapy

Here I was only a few weeks after being told that I had cancer in my leg and lungs and my doctor had me lying totally nude on a cold treatment table with ten to fifteen medical students staring at me. I didn't know what was worse, the emotional devastation of the illness or the humility of the treatment. I had to endure getting tiny tattoos on my body where the radiation would be administered. They needed to make a body cast of my entire body so the radiation lined up exactly the same every time for the next three months. I was eighteen years old and extremely modest about my body. I was mortified that no one gave me the consideration to help me feel less embarrassed.

I was in an emotional upheaval from my diagnosis and the added mortification was unbearable. The preparation for the treatment and having male and female students seeing every part of me was worse than the radiation.

Because I was receiving chemo at the same time, I was transported daily by ambulance to the hospital for my daily dose of naked degradation.

There really aren't a whole lot of words to describe chemotherapy. Just the mention of the treatment gives the average person a feeling of terror. Now imagine that terror magnified by one thousand times and that was what this 18-year-old boy lying in a hospital bed was feeling. Everything I had ever heard or seen on TV about chemo was a horror story - throwing up, going bald and lying in a bed weak and pale. I was in a state of panic. The previous two days were like a sad, disturbing movie and I couldn't change the channel. There was nowhere for me to turn. The darkness couldn't envelop me; the daylight didn't change the truth. If I was stronger I would have tried to run and if I was weaker I would have tried to die, but I was caught in the middle, consumed by fear and disbelief.

The first few weeks of my treatment were very surreal. Most of it was very confusing; it kept me in a haze. I was grateful for that. The expressions on the faces of my friends and family who came to visit were something I could hardly bear. I was happy to see them, but we were left with so little to say. As far as we were concerned, this was probably the last time we would see each other this side of Heaven. What could they say to someone who was helpless and dying? What could I say to someone who was helpless and living? It was the vulnerability all the way around that left the deepest scars. Saying goodbye to friends who were headed of to college or pursuing other plans in their lives was very difficult. While saying goodbye to my friend Jason I can remember wondering if this was, "Goodbye, I'll see you soon," or was this, "Goodbye, see you in the after life."

These were some very trying conversations, particularly in my weak state.

My sister Mary rushed to California from her home in Arizona. My sister Lisa and her family were already with me because her six-year-old daughter was fighting cancer, too. My older brother Richard was on a mission for the church, so it took him a little while to get home. My other brother Greg came home from college and Larry and Ron, who lived close by, all made it to my bedside to love and support me.

I think the person I felt worst for was Genni, my baby sister. When my treatments began, the entire family suffered from my cancer. There were no more daily routines, family dinners, school programs or sporting events. Every day was about throwing up, high fevers, low immune systems and sadness. When Genni would go to school, she was bombarded with questions from my friends who were in her class. The questions were always about how I was holding up, not about how she was feeling or what she was going through. She took a back seat to Kasey, who received a lot of attention because she was my long-suffering girl friend.

That year, my parents and siblings forgot Genni's birthday. It broke my heart when I found out she went through those things and she never complained one time. It gave me an unbreakable bond with her that we will share forever.

After a few months of my chemo, I could see the effects this lifestyle was having on Kasey. She was faithful to visit me. She always smiled while we were together, and she kept up a wonderful front. Inside I could tell she was as emotionally drained as the rest of us. I had to make a very tough decision about our future. We shared a special bond that I would never forget, but the unspoken truth was that she needed to stop coming to visit me and to start getting on with her life. She was still in high school, and had so many memories to make and fun things to experience. I didn't want the memories of her senior year to consist of bedpans, IV drips and constant worry.

All of the lessons about doing the right thing that my parents had instilled in me when I was younger were being tested. I wanted to choose to keep her heart safe, even though it meant my own would break. It was horrible enough for one teenager to live through this nightmare. Why should two kids be dragged into adulthood before it was time?

Although Kasey outwardly fought me on my decision, I knew deep down she was feeling the same things I was. How could she continue to keep up the schedule and emotional turmoil of a boyfriend with cancer? Her schoolwork and social life had suffered. She looked tired, and although she never said it, it was time for her to start living again.

Our break up actually made us closer friends. I never really stopped loving her and she never made me feel guilty for the break up. From that point on when I talked to her I could ask what she was up to and how she was feeling. Our relationship took on a different tone and I was learning to live with it.

I was struggling with the question of whether or not another girl could ever be attracted to me or love me. I felt ugly and undesirable. I didn't want someone to feel sorry for me or be with me for who I used to be. It was Lauren who spent hours and days at my bedside. She had lost her mother to this horrible disease and had a good understanding of where I was coming from.

My boring routine consisted of going to the hospital for two days, getting zapped, then coming home until I felt well enough to go back the next month. About eight months into that schedule, a few buddies that I used to hang out with started coming around. I couldn't do much but watch TV and play video games, but they didn't seem to mind.

Two of my closest friends were Ryan Beck and Seth Boyle. I became closer to them after my high school classmates left for college. Ryan was a year behind me in school; Seth was the same age as me and went to college close to home. They understood that a teenager still lived somewhere inside this weak frame of skin on bones. On occasion they would break me out of my house and we would go for a ride to see friends or just be anywhere but inside the four walls of my living room. Ryan understood the most that I not only lost my health; I lost everything I was. My body that I worked so hard to keep fit was a skeleton. My hair was almost gone and my face was unrecognizable. I could no longer meet the guys for a pick up game of basketball, or a few sets of weightlifting at the gym. Even mud football, which was one of my favorite fun things, wasn't an option for me. My life literally revolved around taking my next breath and getting through the next five minutes without wishing I could die to escape the pain.

It was Ryan and Seth who could see how emotionally devastating it was to lose my hair. Seth tried to ease my burden by shaving his own head down to the scalp so I wouldn't feel out of place being bald. I considered that to be that epitome of friendship.

Seth, Ryan and Jason decided to find a way to turn the tables on the pain I suffered and laugh at it instead. We broke out of my house, went to the local grocery store and I proceeded to act like a lunatic. I was holding my head, making faces and weird noises. Then, as a small group of people gathered, I grabbed a handful of hair and pulled it from my scalp. This caused more than a few people to run away in horror. We would just laugh and they would get me home before my parents found out about the commotion I caused when I left the house.

During one of my ever-boring stays in the hospital for pneumonia, a frequent side effect of chemotherapy, I was lonely, sick, tired, sad, and afraid. Ryan walked in to visit me. He knew by the look on my face that I had a plan. Three weeks in the hospital bed had gotten to me, so I spoke to my nurse that morning about getting a day pass to leave the hospital for a few hours. He said that maybe he could arrange it as soon as I felt well enough. I had a different time frame in mind. That night after everyone left, we escaped. I didn't really have a plan. I just wanted to be free. I unhooked my IV and headed out the door.

We hopped in the car and headed to a friend's house. It felt like old times. I talked to a few people that I went to school with, and for a moment, was able to forget my gruesome circumstances and the health risk I had just put myself in. I had some fun, and I was sure no one would ever find out. When we returned we found out that our prank had repercussions beyond my good time. My nurse had been searching the entire hospital grounds for me. He stayed hours after his shift was over, and I most likely caused him to lose his job. I felt awful and knew I had to make things right. I not only had to plead my case so my parents didn't disown me, but my nurse's case also. It was going to be a while before I pulled another prank like that. (Or until this one blew over; which ever came first.) Shortly after that night, the doctors agreed to teach me to administer my own antibiotics and sent me home for the remainder of my treatments. This arrangement was much better for my mental health. It wasn't the last time I would ignore doctor's orders. I just knew that my stubbornness and road trips were helping keep me alive.

Once I was home, we went on an escapade that turned out to be a little more serious, but also a blessing to the rest of my life. I forced Seth and Ryan to "kidnap" me from my house and take me for a ride. They reluctantly agreed, so we drove for a little while talking and listening to the radio. When we stopped on the side of the road, I saw a brick wall nearby and I decided to climb on it to see what was on the other side. The only thing I found was a mouthful of dirt, and a broken leg. We panicked. I knew I was in big trouble this time. I was supposed to be home resting, and now there was no way to quietly sneak back into the house undetected.

They rushed me to the hospital, and after a few hours I was under the knife to have my bone repaired with a metal rod inserted to help the healing process.

It was during the surgery that my doctor performed a procedure to check on the progress of the tumor that he was radically treating for almost a year. The results were shocking. Although my lungs had made progress, the tumor on my leg looked as though they never started treatment. All of my suffering had been for nothing. No progress had been made. The radiation therapy had only managed to weaken the bone, causing it to break when I fell. We were back to square one. All of those humiliating days of lying naked on a treatment table, with tattooed marks on my body, in front of fifteen to twenty medical students, were for nothing. What did they learn? The same thing that I did; no one had the answer or cure for my disease.

This news caused a huge emotional setback for me. I was clinging by a thread to any hope of living and now I was being told that all of my intense suffering, pain, and the ravaging of my family were to no avail. How could this be? What were my options? I was not ready to die. I knew that all of the nights of excruciating pain when I asked God to take me home to Heaven I hadn't really wanted to die. I could not be the one to hurt my parents by leaving them. I wanted to follow my dreams. I wanted to have a chance to sing. I wanted to be healthy and get married and have a family of my own. I was just a kid. We prayed that there would be another option. The next few days were a frantic search for answers.

A barrage of phone calls, research, and medical inquiries were made on my behalf. Finally, my doctor came to me with one last ditch effort. It was a form of chemotherapy that would bring me as close to death as a human can get without actually taking a last breath.

It would take another year, and make the previous year of treatments seem like a day at the beach. My hospital stays would be longer, my "bounce back time" between visits would be grueling, and I would be experiencing extreme pain as the cancer was being fought off. We had many discussions about the repercussions of this treatment. One side effect was the damage it could cause to my nervous system, which is why today I have only a little feeling in my hands and feet. I even lost complete control of my jaw at times. It would open wider and wider uncontrollably until I thought my head would tear in two. That was scary! At one point I was asked if I wanted to freeze my sperm for future use. No one ever explained how important the decisions I made at this time would be to my future, if I did survive. I could not see past the end of a day let alone past my twenties. My future was never really considered; the options were given only to satisfy the proper paper work. Any discussions never lasted more than a few minutes. What choices did I really have? I had to keep fighting. There was no way to prepare my family for my death. My mom and dad had given up everything they considered "normal." Genni's life was a nightmare, and I knew that I hadn't reached my destiny as a man.

I signed the papers to approve an experiment that would either kill me or kill the disease. This time next year there would be a victory. I prayed it would be mine.

The Poster

My favorite mode of transportation in high school was a Kawasaki Ninja motorcycle. I loved to ride because I felt free as the wind blew into my face and I could feel the speed of the air against my chest. My sister Genni realized how much I must have missed those days while I was sick and she brought me a poster of a motorcycle to keep on the wall. It was a simple picture of a man riding. The bike was similar to the one I owned during high school. It seemed no matter what problems I faced I could jump on that motorcycle and ride to clear my mind.

Ironically, this was the time that I needed to ride more than ever, but my physical condition left me too weak to even consider it. In fact, during one conversation with my doctors, it was mentioned that I would probably never ride again. So I resorted to the next best thing. I would literally project myself into the poster, and in my mind I would ride for hours. I would visit familiar streets and cruise down country roads. I directed my attention toward my imaginary trips and promised myself that I would ride again on a new motorcycle as soon as I beat this thing.

There is no real way to measure how much the kindness and priceless treasure like a poster actually contributed in saving my life, but in my heart and spirit I am confident to say that my survival rests in the hearts and hands of everyone that took special care and time to visit me. Every visit from family and friends or the people from the Make-A-Wish Foundation added to my source of strength and hope. There were many occasions that family and friends may have said an encouraging word or brought me a certain gift that had a huge impact on my survival that day or week. What Genni thought was just a reminder of my healthy days in the past was actually a symbol of what I wanted to live for in my future; the feeling of the wind and freedom and riding as fast as I could away from the memories of the Hell I was in. Most times my visitors would leave my side never knowing how they kept my spirit alive when my body wanted to die. I owed each of them a part of my life. A poster helped carry me through.

David Foster

Four months into my chemo I was laying in my bed and a woman from the Make-A-Wish Foundation came to visit me. She asked me what I would wish for if I had the opportunity. At that point I felt a twinge of fear because I thought to myself that these wishes are for dying children. I still wanted to hope I would live. It was later I found out that the wishes were for children with life-threatening medical conditions of many types. I felt a little better after that discovery. My six-year-old niece who had also battled cancer had gone to Disney Land so I was very happy to get the opportunity because I assumed these wishes were for much younger children. I thought about it for a long time. It was harder than one would imagine, making a wish that required leaving the security of a hospital room or my parents' living room couch. I had grown accustomed to being a hermit.

I thought for a while and mentioned a few different people I would like to meet - Barry Manilow, Billy Joel, or the San Diego Chargers. However, right as our visit was ending I remembered David Foster. David was a music producer in Hollywood that was involved in making a lot of the songs I loved the most. There were many times in my life that music helped me through emotional lows and added to the excitement of the highs. It seemed that whenever a song on the radio or a movie theme song touched me, the credits would include David Foster. Many of my road trip daydreams had me singing songs that were connected to David. As she was leaving my room I blurted out his name. She asked who David was, and said she would try to hunt him down. If my life was going to be cut short, I wanted to meet him, if only to thank him for his music and its impact on my life.

The next thing I knew, my parents and Genni and I were flying to Los Angeles to go to David's studio. I was 18 and had never flown on a plane before. I was a little nervous but happy at the same time. Everything seemed so surreal. I didn't know what I wanted to say to David. I had no idea what he was told about me, or why he thought I wanted to meet him. Of course, I needed to worry about everything that might go wrong and to feel awkward. Worry was my old friend.

As we walked into David's studio I felt like I was on a movie set. Everything about his studio was just as I imagined it; there were hundreds of gold and platinum records aligning the walls, awards and plaques hung everywhere, and the musical equipment was beyond my comprehension. There were Grammy Awards on the tables where the rest of us would have put a family portrait. David went out of his way to invite James Pankow from the group *Chicago* to be there because he knew they were my favorite group.

David worked his magic, taking the tracks and making them sound like a song that was ready for the radio. We sat and listened for hours.

Up to this point in my illness I felt the life leaving my body little by little every day. As I watched him work and saw the love in his eyes for what he was doing, I could feel life and hope come flooding back to me.

When it came time for a break, David pulled me aside and asked me straight out if I was going to die. I told him that the odds were against me, but I was really trying not to die. His simple question made a deep impact in my heart. I knew people for a long time that never asked me that question, but he just blurted it out and caught me off guard. I found something curiously energizing about that. He asked if we could keep in touch. I assured him that I would keep him updated with my progress.

David and my dad formed a strong bond that day. They both had lost their fathers at an early age, and found a few other things in common that made them feel very comfortable with each other. Many times over the next year David called to talk to Dad to check up on me. I went to visit him two or three more times as my chemo progressed.

I considered David to be a person that I could talk to and not have to hide my fear or pain. He was very up front with me about death and never made me feel as though I had to sugarcoat my feelings to protect him from the cruel truth about my cancer. I was just a friend who happened to have cancer. That openness and reality was refreshing for me. It seemed that whenever I needed a pick me up, David would call to check up on me. The Make-A-Wish Foundation had a huge impact on my survival. The strength and blessing I received that day truly helped to save my life.

I was so excited the night that I returned from my visit with David; I wanted to call Kasey to share my experience with her. Our friendship had become close enough again since our mutual break up, we started talking about more personal things, and I was sure she would be happy for me.

When she answered the phone I felt a distance in her voice. She seemed to be less excited for me than I would have expected. She had known about my admiration and respect for David and what meeting him meant to me. I was almost afraid to ask her what was happening, but I did anyway. At that point she told me that she had been seeing another boy, and that they were going steady. My world came crashing down around me. In the midst of the fight of my life, I was faced with the reality that everyone else's life was going on as usual. I was the only one stuck in the mode of living one minute at a time. Kasey could see her future; she really did have an entire lifetime of memories to make. All of the reasons I saw necessary to let her go were still true. I just wasn't ready to face it. My heart sank, my hoped left me, I cried. My day went from the highest of highs to the lowest of lows within an instant. How unfair that I was fighting to stay alive and being flooded with the idea that I didn't have anything to live for.

With no clear motive or reason in my mind I went directly to my medicine case and took pills - lots of pills. I think I just wanted to fall asleep so the pain would stop.

I was not ready for another loss, and although I was the one who initiated the break up with Kasey, I knew I only did it to be fair to her. I was tired of worrying about fair. I wanted to start worrying about me. I was in pain, I was lonely, I was scared, and I was without hope. I was tired of people saying how strong I was. I didn't want to be the strong one anymore.

I just wanted to get the help I so desperately needed.

The Ward

The next morning, my mother found me slumped over the edge of my bed. She then saw the open bottle of pills scattered along the floor and next to my leg. Through my mental fog I could hear the sounds of panic, fear and sorrow. My mother immediately called my oncologist who explained to her that I had taken only enough pills to result in a very bad headache, but to bring me in for my regularly scheduled chemo the next morning and he would take a look at me.

This time my check-in was a bit different. This time I was not treated like poor Kevin with cancer, fighting off another fever, or immune system deficiency problem.

This visit began with me being transported to another facility and admitted into the psych ward for evaluation. The doctors considered my actions as a threat to my own well being and took them very seriously. I spoke for hours to a psychiatrist who wanted to help me uncover the reasons for my depression. I had fought depression and manic highs most my life. Now I was sick and didn't know if I was going to live or die. Of course I was depressed! I didn't need a doctor to explain that one. It wasn't enough that I had been battling cancer for months and so weak I could hardly walk, or that every other week I had to be pumped full of deadly drugs that were ironically keeping me alive, or the fact that the girl I loved just told me she had another boyfriend. This doctor wanted to dig deeper and deeper still.

What I revealed to him was what had plagued my innermost private thoughts since the day I found out I had cancer. I felt as though God was punishing me for becoming sexually active outside the bonds of marriage. That teaching was impressed upon me from such a young age, and my parents were so sure of its importance, that I was feeling extremely guilty for not living up to that moral standard. Kasey and I had crossed a line and I couldn't deal with the fact that I got cancer and she got a new boyfriend. My pain and guilt were so deeply seeded that I could no longer bear the burden.

My honest confession was the beginning of a long series of counseling sessions while I was having my chemo treatments. It was also the beginning of long discussions between Mom and Dad and I. My parents were devastated that I believed that my cancer was a punishment from God. It took them by complete surprise. They never wanted the faith we shared as a family to cause pain. The goal was a better life, not guilt and despair. I guess my tendencies toward worrying and my desire to please them somehow twisted the truths they were trying to teach me.

I had a long road ahead of me, but this time I was not only fighting cancer, depression was added to the battle. The road to recovery had just gotten longer.

Everything about my treatments changed after that night. I had a psychiatric counselor visit me every time I was in the hospital. I was put on anti-depressant drugs, and I was sinking into a hole that I felt would fall in on top of me and bury me alive. The cancer treatment was wreaking havoc with my body and the depression medicine was messing with my mind.

Nights: Something Left To Do

Being sick was always worse at night. Sometimes I was so sick I prayed that my visitors would just go away and let me sleep. I couldn't keep my eyes open. I felt horrible and truthfully, sometimes I didn't want to be around anyone. Other times I felt differently. There were so many nights when I wished my visitors would never leave. I cherished anyone who was the last one at my bedside. Some of my guests were people I hardly even knew. They came to see me because they went to my school or knew my parents. I was always thankful for the caring that accompanied them. Some visitors were my dearest friends who knew how being cooped up and inactive was gnawing away at my spirit.

Nighttime was the great equalizer. I cherished any person that gave me reason to keep the light on and any voice that would keep speaking to me.

There was something about the darkness that brought out my fear. Of all of the demons I had to wrestle with in my life, it was always the ones that visited during the night that could fight the longest. I always thought it was because they brought sadness and guilt along as back up. When one got tired another could jump right in and take over.

One night in particular stands out in my mind as a life-altering event. My dad was asleep on a bed next to me in my hospital room. I was extremely ill and groggy from the pain. I felt an eerie presence in my room impressing upon me that I should give up my fight and die. Almost audibly it was reminding me that this fight was much bigger than I was. What ever it was had an evil that made a chill run down my spine. I tried to scream, but the terror I was feeling was blocking the sound from escaping my mouth. I was paralyzed. Finally, I managed to eke out a yelp that awoke my dad. He came to my bedside to comfort me, but could immediately see the panic on my face. I told him, "He's trying to get me. He's trying to get me." When Dad asked who was trying to get me I told him it was the Devil. He held me and told me everything was going to be all right. He had no idea what had just happened. After we settled back into bed, the same thing happened again two more times, each time becoming more and more intense. My Dad came to my rescue again. The third time I asked him to pray with me. For every prayer he prayed, I doubled his pleas in my heart, which helped to ease my fear. I never experienced a supernatural evil before. It was real and it was beyond explanation.

After he returned to bed and fell asleep, I had another visit, but this time it was pure peace. I was not feeling any pain; I had no fear, and didn't have a need to call to my father. I felt safe. I wasn't sure if it was a visit from an angel or God Himself, but whoever it was reassured me that cancer was not my destiny. I had a much more important destiny. In a quiet tender voice I heard the words, "You have something left to do." That was exactly the moment I knew I would live. I didn't know how long, but I knew that this was not the night I would die. I was certain that I needed to keep fighting if I ever wanted to find out what my purpose in life was and why I was still alive. If I indeed had something else to do I wanted to know what it was, and why I was important enough to get two extremely different visits in the middle of the same night.

The next morning I never spoke a word of what had happened. I was sure my dad thought I was having a reaction from my medication. I didn't feel the need to try to explain or persuade him or anyone else to believe any differently. I was convinced that I knew the truth. I felt that I was somehow let in on the "real truth." Only living would allow me to find out what my true destiny was. I vowed in my heart to search for my destiny until I was sure I found it. I hoped that someday it would be revealed to me.

Round Two

The events that occurred in my life during my second year of treatment were beyond my comprehension. I reached my all time lowest point and I experienced an all-time highest point in my nineteen years.

The effects of the chemo this time went beyond torture. When my doctors told me that I would come close to death they weren't exaggerating. Within a month of the first cycle I was convinced I would not survive. I started to deal with the fact that I was going to die. I accepted it. I wondered how I could have prayed for victory just weeks before and now wished I could just blow away. The hardest part for me still was watching the faces of the friends and family that visited me. I felt so sad for them. I wished I could comfort their pain.

Every time I had to go for another round of chemo I would start to get sick before I got into the car to leave the driveway.

The ride to the hospital was like slow torture. The smell when I entered the building started my body's gag reflex and I would throw up before I got through the lobby. By the time I reached the pediatrics or cancer ward I was already so sick I needed a few hours of recovery time before I could start my actual treatments. There are certain smells and sounds that go hand in hand with cancer and chemotherapy that only a cancer patient can understand.

Most of the time I was able to stay in the pediatrics ward of the hospital, which was a blessing for me. The nurses and caregivers there seemed to have more kindness and there was a sense of hope as compared to the few times I had to be in the adult cancer ward. I guess there is something that brings out compassion when a child suffers. The nurses used to fight over who would be my caregiver for the week that I would be there, partly because I didn't require constant care. Unlike most of the other patients, I didn't require spoon feedings, diapers, or the immediate care that a small child would. Although I felt terrible, I was able to be alone and still with my thoughts. At that time, I daydreamed a lot about becoming a singer and what it would be like to have an audience while I sang my favorite songs. It was daydreaming that helped me through my living nightmare. It was the hope of becoming a singer that kept me alive.

When I was in the middle of a week in the hospital being pumped full of toxic waste or lying on my parents couch trying not to throw up, I would lose my ability to fight. I would struggle to survive for five minutes, only to find that five more awaited me with even more pain and suffering. Visualizing my success as a singer was the only thing that kept me sane. I would lie there and let my mind transport me to a performance or road trip. I could close my eyes and imagine every aspect of being on stage singing to my fans or on the bus writing songs with my musician friends. I would envision fine details like what I would wear, what cities we would play, and names of the songs I would sing and to whom I would dedicate each one to. I became so engrossed in my dreams that before I knew it an hour might have passed. (In chemo time, an hour is equal to an eternity.) There were a few times that I could have just quit and followed the peacefulness of the light on the other side. However, I would always return knowing I couldn't stop fighting yet. I could never fault anyone for following that warmth and peace that comes from the other side. I was so tempted, but it just wasn't my time.

Kelly

Most of the new people I met while I was sick were nurses, doctors, hospital personnel or children who had cancer. My choices were either people who were going to cause me pain, see me naked and helpless, or those that had the same cloud of death hanging over them as I did. That was not such a great beginning to a lasting relationship. I was always hesitant to enter the room of a pediatric cancer patient when I came in for chemo, because I was afraid I would find an empty bed or someone new occupying my old friend's space. I would feel sadness, not only because I lost a friend, but because there were no answers to questions like, "Why am I still alive and they're not?" My odds were just as horrible as his or hers. Or, how much more loss of faith and hope can I take as each one of these children passes on? Still, I found myself becoming attached to another and another after that one. Unfortunately, there was never a shortage of sick children when I went to the hospital.

Sometimes I would go from room to room on the ward and sing for the kids and their families. I would sing, *Please Don't Be Scared*, by Barry Manilow or other songs that helped me through rough times.

On one visit I met Kelly, she was a little girl who was suffering from brain cancer and had already outlived her doctor's prognosis. I immediately felt a bond with her and her parents. Kelly was so strong and brave that despite her ravaged body she was still a bundle of hope and life.

I continued to keep in touch with her family and went to dinner at their home. I even had the privilege of singing the same song I sang for her a few months before at her school talent show. I gleaned incredible courage from Kelly and cherish the lessons she taught me about living every day fully and with hope.

A few months later we lost Kelly. I was devastated, and although her family asked me to sing at her funeral, I was too distressed to bring myself to do it. I sang at funerals before, but this was different and extremely personal. Kelly taught me things that will stay with me for the rest of my life. I think of her often and feel blessed to know I have an angel in my corner.

I visited her grave eight years later to ask for her forgiveness for not singing at her funeral. It was then and only then that my decision stopped eating at me.

Remission

After the second year of my therapy was over, it was time to take more tests to see if we had made any progress on shrinking the cancer. I will never forget the day I received the news that I was in remission. It was surprisingly underwhelming for me. My doctors came into the office, looked me and my parents in the eyes, and told us that the cancer was gone. My mother took a deep breath of relief, my dad hugged me joyfully, and I just stood there. I was in a state of disbelief about my remission combined with disbelief that I wasn't going to die.

I had spent the last two years of my life preparing to die and fighting to live. When I got the news that I would live I was actually caught off guard.

What was I supposed to do now? I didn't have the strength to do manual labor; I didn't have the opportunity to go to college with my friends. I was taking anti-depressants that put crazy thoughts in my head. I felt that I had lost my appearance to my treatments. In some strange way, I was more defeated by living than by dying. I had to accept death as a way of getting ready for the fight. I had to be willing to emotionally and mentally give up my life in order to not be distracted when trying to save it. Learning to live again would prove to be just as hard or even harder.

So here I was with a second chance at life. I should be jumping with joy, shouting praises from the rooftops, on my knees thanking the Lord for sparing my life. Instead I had this sinking feeling deep inside my soul. After being childlike for so long, depending fully on others for my every need, spending all of my time in hospitals, recovering from surgery after surgery, poked and prodded by doctors and nurses and living in a sick bed, now I was expected to move forward. I couldn't remember what forward was. For the past two years of my life, time stood still while everyone else kept going. Everyone else had changed and made progress. The only thing that changed for me was that the cancer was gone. The pain was still there. My body was still weak. I couldn't remember what feeling normal was like. I would have to give a new definition to normal and I didn't like the things this new normal came with. I was still nauseous in the mornings; my leg was useless except to walk really slowly, my knee could not bend and it hurt a lot.

My doctors assured me that my hair would grow back thicker than it ever was. It wasn't long before I realized that would not be the case for me. It grew back thin and patchy and I looked like I had the mange. I don't know why I was so emotionally devastated by the thought of never having my hair back, but I think it was the idea of returning to normal that I wanted so badly after two years of being totally hairless.

My parents decided that we would take a family portrait to celebrate my survival and when we were lining up for the photographer he said to me, "You must be the oldest. You stand here." Of course being second to the youngest I was devastated. I immediately went in search of every conceivable hair replacement system available, which was very limited at that time. I tried spray-on hair and a wig, neither of which were any less conspicuous than my own troubled locks.

I was consumed with the thought that every woman that I passed was wondering what was wrong with me and my pathetic hair.

Finally, after my self-confidence was at an all time low, I took a razor and shaved every hair from my head. I immediately felt better. I was used to being bald and deciding to stay that way. It was one way to solve the problem. I didn't have to worry if people were looking at me and wondering what was wrong with me. Now

I was just a guy who *chose* to shave his head.

Several months after my last treatment, I was still in terrible pain. I was taking pain medication and depression medication, neither of which was helping very much. Then one day I found a lump on my right leg in exactly the same place the cancer had attacked my left leg. My heart sank. I went to the hospital for my post treatment appointment and was told that because my treatments had ended and I was now an adult, I couldn't see the pediatric doctors that I was comfortable with. I was sent to the adult oncology clinic for the first of my many check-ups. I was very concerned that the cancer had come back, so I immediately told the new doctor about the lump I had found. He looked me straight in the eye and said, "I think you are so worried about the cancer returning that you are feeling things that aren't there." I couldn't believe my ears. I was exactly in the same situation as I was in high school with doctors telling me that my pain and concerns were all in my head. I left that clinic and decided that if I were to get sick again I would be able to tell and would go about finding a new doctor on my own. I never went back to that clinic again.

The next year was a challenge for my family and me. I started drinking to mask my pain, and hung around the house watching TV. I was also taking morphine every day for pain. I couldn't get a grip on what I had been through. My family had made so much sacrifice. I had spent years dreaming of things that I thought would never come true, and now I felt I had no purpose. The anti-depressant drugs sure didn't live up to their name. I was in a deep, dark tunnel and couldn't see the light of day.

I still dreamed of music and performing, but since I didn't need the dreams to get me through the fear of cancer or dying; they seemed to lose their luster. I never

thought that singing would be my future.
I didn't really care that much anymore.

It's Always Something

Early on in my treatments it was necessary to have an IV port surgically placed under the skin on my left upper chest area.

Anyone who has spent an extended amount of time in the hospital knows first hand that veins and arteries can only withstand so much abuse before they just stop working.

This port worked like an outlet for the treatments or emergency drugs that were necessary for my hospital visits. The procedure to administer it was simple enough - a small incision and a line running directly into my artery. This procedure made it easy for nurses or doctors to "plug in" directly to my bloodstream without having to find a vein (which after months of treatments would have been impossible.)

The port proved to be very successful during my 20 months of treatment. I experienced less pain because of it.

Now that I was in remission, the doctors felt that I no longer needed the port and scheduled my visit to have it removed. The original incision would have to be reopened and the line gently pulled out of my artery.

As I lay motionless on the table, the line was being pulled out when it suddenly broke off and flipped into my heart. Now the situation was a bit different. If the line moved at all in any direction it could kill me. My simple procedure had turned into emergency, life-saving surgery. It was necessary for me to be awake during the entire thing so I just prepared myself for what was coming next.

I was assured that it would be quick and easy. By inserting a wire into my groin area and following the arterial path to my heart, the doctor could hook the tube and pull it free. Everything was going as planned until it was time to pull the tube out. After being inside my chest for so long, the tube actually grew attached to the artery and was stuck.

The plan was to pull very hard and release it. With every tug, the pain was becoming more and more intense. One last tug was all it took for the tube to loosen and flip even further into my heart. With that, monitor alarms, panic and expressions of fear took over the room. I was gripped with pain and felt myself slipping into unconsciousness. Just at that point, the doctor slapped me very hard across the face in an attempt to keep me awake. I was shocked, in pain and beyond fearful.

I remember more doctors running into the room, and as I drifted in and out of awareness, I felt as though my spirit was leaving my body and watching the entire scenario from above myself on the table.

I was rushed by ambulance to a cardiac hospital and I heard things being said like, "We will have to crack his chest open," and "I can't lose this one." In my mind I was thinking that he better not lose me. I have come too far to lose the battle in such a crazy way. As we got to the hospital, I heard someone say that he was going to give the arterial wire one more shot because this guy was too young to have his chest opened. At that point I passed out.

When I woke up it was over. I didn't have to have open-heart surgery after all. The last shot at the wire had worked.

It wasn't easy finding a bright spot in that situation, but I remember my first thought was how great it was that I didn't have a huge scar running the length of my chest.

This situation was one more piece of evidence that I had more to accomplish in my life and that I was being spared. I was curious to find out why.

Rebuilding a Body and Soul

The first step to my destiny was to repair my leg as best as it could be. I couldn't put on my own sock or shoe; sit in the back seat of a car or anything else that required bending my knee. The radiation had basically cooked the muscle in my leg until it would no longer stretch. I needed two surgeries and a painful two-week stretching treatment to help the process. I endured them with the hope of regaining some sort of normalcy in my very abnormal life. I went through another fight to repair the effects of cancer and I again took home the victory.

Although I won back the use of my leg, something was still tormenting my soul. I was still allowing small matters to become huge dragons in my life. I wondered if I would be able to find a girlfriend or wife who would want a man that could never have children, walked with a limp, could never be athletic, have a tough time making a living, and who had scars all over his body? I was consumed with these questions. I also had a very bad case of survivor's guilt. I would lie awake wondering why so many kids on the ward had lost their fight and died. Why I was spared and not them? I began to question my mortality and would do reckless things, like driving very fast when I was behind the wheel of my car.

Then one day I started doing something that I never dreamed was in me to do. I began cutting myself on my arm and chest with a razor and a knife. I convinced myself that the pain of the cut would ease the pain I was feeling inside. I was so preoccupied with cleaning up the blood and tending the new cut that I would forget my problems for those few minutes. But there was one problem with my new coping method. It didn't fix anything. Surely you can lie, cheat and steal to avoid your problems but now you only have more problems. I still had my other problems and now on top of them I had scars on my chest and arms that I had to explain to my mom. When she realized what I was doing, and saw my self-inflicted wounds, it broke her heart. It was the look in her eyes that made something change in my heart. I realized at that point that the lie I had convinced myself of was just a bunch of bull. I was not feeling any better by cutting myself, it was not a great coping mechanism and I was not the same Kevin I used to be before my illness. Now that I was going to be living a long life I knew I had to pull myself together and start climbing out of this deep darkness I was in. I prepared myself for another fight. This time it was a battle to win back the rest of my life.

As time went on I was still on daily pain and depression medications. I could not function as the same person I was before my illness. That boy was long gone. I couldn't put my finger on the exact direction I was heading and I wasn't sure of my destiny. I struggled with so many questions and not enough answers. I felt alone and helpless. I just wanted to be back to the Kevin I was so many years before. I needed to find a way to start over, but the thing I needed to do most was to stop taking the drugs that the doctors had prescribed and get free to live again. I had to find out what was worse, the pain or the side effects of the many drugs.

I made a drastic (and not so intelligent) decision. I quit all of my narcotics on the same day! I imagined it would be difficult, but I never actually comprehended how life threatening it would be. In a way, I'm glad I didn't know. The only thing I was certain of was that I had reached the end of my rope of having crazy thoughts, feeling lethargic about life and not knowing what to do next.

I decided to stop the anti-depressants, the pain meds and the drinking all at once, cold turkey! At this point I was on methadone (a form of heroin) for my pain. This wasn't going to be easy.

What came next was grueling, painful and inhumane, but I was in control of my destiny for the first time in years. To me, this move was a positive one. Despite my agony, I could almost envision a ray of sunshine peeking out from the dark clouds.

For the next twenty-eight days, my life was exactly what you would see in a movie about a drug addict going cold turkey. Shaking, convulsions, sweating, throwing up, and insomnia were typical behavior for my level of addiction. My body was going to fight me every step of the way, but my will to fight back was stronger. I lay on my parents living room floor day after day trying to survive, promising myself that if I wasn't better by morning I would go to the hospital. Finally, on day 28 I kept that promise to myself and went to see my doctor. He couldn't believe what I had done and was relieved to see that the process didn't kill me. He immediately had me admitted so I could finish the self-inflicted journey I started on my own almost a month before. As much as I hated hospitals I had to admit it felt good to be taken care of for a few days. I completed my quest and was now determined to get my life in order. I was on the hunt for the Kevin I left behind almost three years before. Although I was clean for a while, I would continue to struggle with the balance of pain relief and a functioning lifestyle. The reality of chronic pain is not feeling like me while on the medication but without it, the pain makes me crazy. It's the hardest balancing act to pull off and most of us can't.

Building a Dream

Now that I was clean from the medications, had a knee that could bend and a bald head by choice, my life began to take on some order. I was slowly regaining more of myself. My mind was becoming clearer and my ambitions were no longer clouded in a dense fog. I started to believe that I really had something special inside me and the people around me were starting to see my potential as well.

Along with my new clean and sober life came my re-ignited pursuit of a record deal. Once again I remembered my love for music and all of the times in the past I ached to live the life of a star. I wasn't quite clear about the proper procedures to "go for it," but I was compelled to chase it. I would sing most of the days from dawn until dusk and the feedback was flattering. I heard comments like, "You sing that song as good as the real guy," and "Wow, Garth doesn't do it any better than you." Unfortunately, those comments were the crux of the problem. My ability to sing cover tunes as well as the original singer didn't mean anything to record labels. They wanted to hear original songs that were as great as cover tunes.

I knew that I wasn't up to that standard of writing, so I set out to find a co-writer. That was the first piece of a very intricate puzzle. However, before I actually met anyone, my brother Richard told me about a college friend of his that had a similar dream to mine. He wanted to be a famous songwriter. I'd had too many experiences with "coincidences" in the past to ignore this twist of fate. I flew to Utah to meet Eric Bunch.

We immediately hit it off. I liked his songs; he liked my voice. We used his very simple recording system to put a song to tape and knew we had to work together in some capacity. We just had to figure out how.

I returned to California and enrolled in music and recording classes at the community college. There was no doubt in my mind that the things I learned would serve me well in the future. One day in class we started to study home studios. Our assignment was to design a studio from top to bottom, complete with total cost and equipment. Once I saw the results on paper, I instantly knew that this was the next piece of the puzzle.

With the help (and garage) of my dad and Richard, we started to plan out Sharpsounds Studio. I was overwhelmed that they believed in me enough to invest money and muscle into building a recording studio. We sent Eric the money he needed to get the equipment to start laying music tracks. We did construction, soundproofing, and equipment installation. Everything was timed so the studio would be done in time for Eric's visit to record my vocals.

Finally, after weeks of hard work and a lot of sweat, we finished. By the time Eric arrived, I was exhausted. I was almost too sick to record, but we pressed on. Sickness was not going to interfere with my new life. It had taken too much from me already. I was in control this time. We worked in the studio for 5 days straight without more than a few hours of sleep. We recorded a demo that I could use to shop a deal and also to audition for a show on TNN called *You Can Be A Star*. It was the country version of *Star Search* and I desperately wanted to be on it. We had to work tirelessly to make the audition deadline and we did it. I was so proud of that first tape. We sent it everywhere and to any one we knew that might help us.

The feedback was excellent. Our family and friends loved it. We landed an audition and interest from a small label in Florida

Our passion to succeed was unstoppable. Eric and I knew we were on the right path; our dream was becoming a reality to us. The more we spoke it and told others about it, the more real it became. We were songwriters and I was a singer! The only thing left to do was to let the entire world know it! I had to find the courage to play it for David Foster and to get his advice. I wanted to do it in person, which was very scary to say the least. After meeting and turning down the offer from the small label out of Florida, I thought the offers would just keep coming, they didn't. It would be two long years before the next real offer would come along.

Showcase

My newfound zest for life brought me on many new adventures. I took a job in a mortuary singing for funerals. I joined a local band, sang at "Great America" (a theme park in Northern California) and I even delivered singing telegrams. I wanted to do anything I could that would allow me to sing. Even though many months, even a year had gone by since Eric and I made our demo tape, in my mind I was going for it.

My pursuit for a record deal was a state of mind for me. As long as I continued on with my dream I would be okay. I kept on singing. I was even given the opportunity to make an album locally with a musician, Steve Sitton, who put a lot of time and money into the belief of my career.

Then one day, Jaymes Foster from David Foster's office called and asked if I was still pursuing a deal. She had found my demo tape that I had sent almost two years previous in a box that was slated for the garbage. She took a listen to see if there was anything in there worth a first or second listen. David was starting a label and seeking talent.

One thing led to another and before I knew what was happening, I was in Los Angeles meeting with Chris Farren and auditioning for Kyle Lehning from Asylum records! I had never experienced anything like it before. I thought my audition for the summer theatre was scary; I had no idea how frightening the big time could be.

Here I was, having had one rehearsal with unfamiliar musicians, no audience, in a tension-filled room of industry big wigs. My family was back at home and David Foster had put his reputation on the line on my behalf. Part of me wanted to go home, but the dreamer in me had been preparing for this day my entire life.

Before we began, David came over and put his hand on my shoulder. His last words of encouragement for me were, "Don't f_ _ _ this up." Those words surely put me at ease!

When the music started, I took a deep breath and at that point I pretended I was on stage in front of the thousands of fans I had imagined all of those nights during chemo. I sang and I gave them what I knew I had in me and I didn't hold anything back. When I finished my first song, the room was filled with dead silence. My heart was pounding in my chest. My mind was like a runaway freight train. "They hated me, I could have done better, and David is going to kill me." Just then I heard the music to my second song begin and there I was again singing like I was the biggest thing to hit the music industry. No one had any reaction, just poker faces and dead silence. I was thinking that I was finished, but I continued on in this same manner until all of the songs were finished.

When I sang my last note, I hopped down off the stage and went to where the refreshments were. Feeling nervous and defeated, I was surprised when Kyle Lehning came up behind me, shook my hand and said, "Let's do this."

I wasn't sure what that meant, but as I glanced over at David and saw that he was smiling, I knew things went well. Then it hit me, I was right in the middle of realizing my biggest dream. I was getting my record deal after all!

I ran out into the back alley and called my parents. I was so excited I didn't want anyone to see me jumping around like a lunatic among the dumpsters and empty crates as I told my father all about every detail of my incredible experience.

The Real Journey Begins

After listening to literally thousands of songs and weeding them down to what we felt was the best of the best, was it time to record.

I remember the first day I went into the studio to record my first album. I was the one who got to be the fan. The best studio musicians available were all there. I asked each of them for an autograph. They looked at me like I was crazy, but I wanted to have memories of this day that I dreamed of for so long throughout my illness. Everyone there was important to me. I even asked the studio assistant who filled the coffee, hot chocolate and snacks to sign an autograph. Long days in the studio concentrating and trying to get everything just right would be unbearable if the coffee and snacks ran out! That assistant was very important to me!

Each time I entered the studio I wanted to be sure that every song I performed was one that I loved and could see myself singing hundreds of times over as though it was the first time. I wanted to make sure that all of the never-ending hours on the road; radio station interviews and concerts would be fresh every time. I always wanted my fans to get my best!

The road to getting fans was the hardest part. Once my first album was finished and everything sounded great, the craziness started. Now it was time to get the radio stations across America to play my first single, "Nobody Knows." I was an unknown artist, the radio programmers didn't know me, and no one ever wants to be first to try out an unknown. I spent months on the road going to radio stations doing interviews and meeting the programmers and DJ's. It was exciting and exhausting at the same time. The radio turned out to be very friendly to me. 105.1 in Sacramento showed their support from the very beginning, even before I had a major label deal. They were the first station to ever play, "Nobody Knows" on the airwaves. The morning team of "Pat and Tom" at KNCI were very good to me then and now. Hearing myself on the radio was a joy that doesn't get any better!

Before I knew it, I was on almost every country radio station and television talk show. I was making guest appearances on TV, doing many live performances, and was nominated for an "Academy of Country Music Award" and "American Music Award." I felt like I had died and gone to Heaven.

The Business of Making Music

When I finally got my record deal I was so excited. I let my mind wander and dream about how much money I was about to make and all of the great things I would be able to afford to do. I was going to be rich! After all if I was going to be on the radio and television and making guest appearances and doing concerts, I should be able to expect the riches to follow, right?

The only thing I had to do was to listen to the advice of my new lawyers and everything would be great. Record contracts are tricky and need to be handled with a keen eye and sharp mind. I was a wide-eyed kid whose dreams were about to come true. The law firm I was referred to was tops in the entertainment field. They represented the top artists in the business. I was told that my contract was "standard" and I trusted them to do a good job for me.

I knew in my heart that money was never a driving force for pursuing my career in music; it was only a great bonus. I simply wanted to sing and record great songs.

I had taken a music business course in junior college, so I thought I would be fairly prepared for what was going on.

I soon learned that the music industry is not something that is learned from a book or from a teacher that never had a record deal.

All of a sudden I was getting advice from people who never had time for me before. New "friends" were coming out of the woodwork and everyone had great ideas for my career. It was all very overwhelming, but on the other hand it was also very exciting to share my good news with the family and friends who were always there believing in me.

When it came time to get down to real business, the record label gave me a thirty-thousand-dollar advance to keep me afloat while I recorded and got ready for touring. I thought that it was very generous of them; my lawyer assured me that it was a standard procedure. I knew I could finally relax and just make a great album.

My attorney had a reputation for being very good, and when I got the bill, I realized that "good" meant expensive. My bill was for $15,000! I could not believe it! I had to pay half of my advance to a lawyer that had spent less than fifteen hours on my "standard" contract.

I immediately started to research other firms to see if I was getting ripped off (which I believed I was) and much to my disappointment, I learned that I was, in fact, paying the going rate for good attorneys representing new artists. That fact didn't make it right, but at least I knew I wasn't alone.

All the artists were making financial sacrifices in one way or another. It was the price for being a part of "the biz." I don't think being "one of the many" having to pay the price made me feel any better, but for the sake of my music, future fans and my family, I went ahead and paid the bill.

I figured it was the record label's money anyway, so why should I be so upset? What I didn't know at the time was that the show biz synonym for "advance" was "loan.' I had to pay back the thirty thousand as well as all other expenses incurred on my behalf for recording, promotion, photos, touring and everything else, before I ever received another dime.

The stakes were so high I knew I had no choice but to succeed. I couldn't afford to be a flop. In some ways I think that experience was a great lesson for the rest of my life. It pushed me to work harder and to go for the gusto. Whatever was going to happen from that point on gave me the opportunity to be one of the very few that would live out this amazing dream.

My experience was the course they should have taught at Junior College. Welcome to Showbiz!

Tattoo

I believe that laughter is truly a healing gift from God. If we can learn to laugh at our own shortcomings, we would be much healthier in mind, body and especially spirit. I usually find several reasons every day to laugh at myself. Mostly because I continually need to be reminded that I really have little to no control over the things that happen in life.

This truth is revealed to me everyday when I take off my shirt and see my reflection in the mirror.

It was a very exciting time when Asylum Records was going to release my first single, "Nobody Knows" to the radio and to the world. I was experiencing days filled with photo shoots, interviews, recording sessions and meetings. My schedule was enough to make my head spin, but I was thrilled by it all. It was during one of those whirlwind days that I came up with the idea that if my song hit

#1 on the charts, that I and a few of my label friends should all get tattoos. Thinking that my chances of going to #1 were about the same as getting struck by lightening, we went ahead and actually signed a contract agreeing that we would each get a tattoo of our choice if the song hit #1 on the Billboard Country Chart. One member of our "scheme team" didn't want a tattoo, so instead signed that he would shave his head!

At the time I signed, I had never been and still wasn't a tattoo kind of guy, but didn't think I had anything to worry about. I was wrong. As the weeks passed and the song climbed the charts, it was exciting on one hand and dreadful on the other. I did not want a tattoo!! In fact, I had nightmares about having to honor my word, not to mention a written contract! After a few weeks, the song hit #1 and before I knew it, I was deciding what I was going to have permanently penned onto my body. The thought was dreadful to me, but my word was my bond.

I came to the decision that I would ask my mother for help. My plan was to kill two birds with one stone. Break the news to her and get her opinion at the same time. I thought that if she had a say in it, the pill would be easier to swallow. I was almost right. My mom is the opposite of anything having to do with the stereotypical tattoo wearer and now her own son would be sporting one. After her initial horror, she slowly became a fountain of ideas. She wanted something that wouldn't embarrass the family, and I wanted something that would stand the test of time. I agonized for weeks over my decision. I had known guys with ex-wives' names permanently on their bodies. This didn't go over too well with the new wives. I would be wearing this decision on my skin for the rest of my life. Just then, as though a light went on in Mom's head, she said, "the Make A Wish logo." Eureka, that was it! I loved that organization. They were there for me when I needed them, and surely that logo would never change. The decision was made, so off I went to honor my contract. I would have a wishbone with the accompanying ribbon tattooed on my chest.

I must admit, after I had the tattoo for a few weeks, it started to grow on me. I was actually proud to bear the logo of Make-A-Wish. Then, a few months later, in true Kevin Sharp style, I received word that due to trademarking issues and the fact that the wishbone represents death in certain cultures, the Make-A-Wish logo was now changed!

I just had to throw up my hands and laugh. It was apparent to me that God's sense of humor is far more refined than my mine will ever be, and if He thinks it's funny then who am I not to laugh!

Now, when things get tough I can look down at my chest and remember that laughter is the best medicine for any situation!

'Til Death Do Us Part

When I was in my teens there were two things I would have bet a million to one that I would never have to deal with; a drug problem was one and divorcing once I was married was the other. I was so into sports and building a healthy body that drugs were never on my radar for social fun, and my religious upbringing didn't leave any wiggle room for divorce. As the saying goes, "Never say never."

I had no idea when I formed those opinions that my life was going to make the twists and turns that found me addicted to pain medications after cancer had damaged my body, nor did I realize that marrying the wrong person could also act like a cancer that damages the soul.

After I battled my drug addiction and things were going well with my music career, I, along with my family, decided the time was right to marry the girl I had been dating for over a year. She was there for me through my struggles, we had the same spiritual beliefs, and both sets of parents gave us their blessings. We agreed it was the right decision at the time.

As we planned our big day, feelings of doubt crept into both of our minds, but neither of us had the courage to say anything. Neither of us wanted to hurt the other, or walk away, so unfortunately our feelings were never voiced until after the wedding. We were both great people who were just not great for each other.

We tried for a year to make it work on the advice of our church bishop, but by then hurt and anger overwhelmed the situation and we both agreed to end our marriage. The divorce was painful for both of us, but in our hearts we knew we were doing what was right.

So here I was, a country music success with a gold album, two #1 radio hits, concerts and fans, living my career dream, and my personal life was a wreck. I kept wondering if I would ever find balance. Would everything ever be good all at once? Does anyone really have it all?

It only took about a year for me to find out that having it all takes on new meaning when you finally meet the person God intended for you from the beginning of time.

I was at the peak of my career, performing at country music's biggest fan event called Fan Fair. All the country music fans from around the world gather in Nashville for a week long festival. All the record labels, artists and musicians come to greet and get to know the fans. It's a crazy time and an honor for artists to be there. I was positioned next to Neal McCoy, who I had met, along with his family at my very first Fan Fair. He was there again with his wife and family who were helping with tee shirts and other souvenirs.

During the first day, I looked over into Neal's booth and saw his wife's sister,

Traci. It was literally love at first sight. She took my breath away. Traci was the girl that my dreams were made of. She was a beautiful brunette with big blue eyes and a smile that stole my heart. I knew she was the blessing that God had for me all along. This time I was going to do everything right and not let her get away.

The more I got to know Traci, the more I loved her. She had been around the music industry enough with Neal to know that it was a hard, bumpy and unpredictable road. The twists and turns wouldn't catch her off guard, she loved country music and we made a great team. It was evident to both of us that we were meant to be together. After many outrageously high cell phone bills and a lot of airline tickets, a year later we were married.

Not long after our honeymoon we experienced our first trial together. I was dropped from my record label. The label was going through many changes and the people I knew there and the ones who championed my efforts were all gone. That meant that I had no more radio support, no more tour support and no more of any of the perks that go along with being under the protection of a record company. It was just me and Traci and my fans.

Although times were tough financially, (a few hit songs doesn't make the artist a millionaire) and emotionally, and we went through another surgery, broken bones and even the devastating loss of Traci's father to cancer, we have remained committed and in love.

Have there been times when either of us had enough cause to walk away? Yes. Have there been times when we thought we couldn't make it? Yes. Do I still think she is the most beautiful woman and biggest blessing in my life? Yes! Do we respect and love each other for better or worse? Absolutely! That is why we are together. We share a pure God-given love for each other that cannot be broken by our circumstances or the state of our careers.

Traci and I have spent six years working things out as they come along. We continue to dream about our goals as a couple and we plan to forge ahead into whatever opportunities come our way and to someday soon start our own little family. I love Traci and am thankful that she never gives up on us. That's what I call balance!

Matthew's Wish

I will always owe a debt of gratitude to the Make-A-Wish Foundation for being another part of the puzzle that saved my life. My visit to meet David Foster was incredible and a dream come true. It was the caring and love of the Foundation staff that touched me and gave me strength to fight back and live.

After I went to Los Angeles to meet David, I wrote a letter of gratitude to the Sacramento chapter and vowed to always be a "wish kid" and gladly do my part to help them whenever I could.

When I wrote that letter, I never dreamed I would be able to live up to that promise, but years later found myself in shock as I learned that a young boy living in his hospital bed as I did eight years before now wished to meet me.

I received a call from my manager saying that a young seven-year-old boy had contacted the Make-A-Wish Foundation and said that, "Nobody Knows" was his favorite song and he wanted to meet the guy who sang it. I wasn't sure he even knew my name and I didn't care! To imagine that my music was helping someone else hold on while they were fighting a horrible disease was unbelievable. Being on the other side of the wish was indescribable to say the least.

The only problem with this wish was that time was against us. Matthew had very little time and I was far away, but the arrangements were made and before I knew it I was on a plane to Houston, Texas to fulfill a wish. It was seven years before that I was on my first plane ride to be the recipient of a wish. Now the circumstances had come full circle.

I suddenly realized what David Foster must have been feeling. What was I going to say to Matthew? Who was I to be someone's wish? Could I live up to what he hears in my music?

There were so many other things a seven-year-old boy could have asked for.

I was unprepared for the feelings that came next. I was greeted at the airport by ladies from the local Foundation and rushed directly to the hospital. We were met by Matthew's parents who couldn't find words to express their gratitude. The entire experience was overwhelming.

I was so wrapped up in the honor, I never prepared for the reality of the situation. As I walked into his room, I could see this fragile child hooked up to every machine that could fit into the room. He was hardly conscious and couldn't speak. As the tears rolled down my face I knew that this experience would change me forever.

As I sat next to him, I watched as a nurse used a suction devise every few minutes to clear his windpipe. I sang, "Nobody Knows" at his bedside and although it was brief, everyone in the room got to see him smile.

I asked to have a moment alone with Matthew and although I could see how loving and wonderful his parents were, I could tell they were having a struggle with letting him go. So many times we make the mistake of allowing our dying loved one to suffer because we don't have the strength to let them go. Sometimes there just isn't a miracle in Heaven and it is simply someone's time to go. In Matthew's case I could see that he was waiting for someone to tell him it was okay to stop fighting. I leaned in and told him that everyone was going to be all right. No one would forget him and everyone would always love him. I told him that I was sick a long time ago too, but for some reason I didn't die. I could sense a peace come over him and I felt peaceful knowing that he understood what I was saying to him. Even though he was a child, he was so smart and so tough and brave.

Matthew passed away just three short days later, but the gift he gave to me will live on in my heart and soul forever. He allowed me to fulfill my promise to the Make-A-Wish Foundation, but more importantly, he allowed me to give encouragement and love to a child that was fighting to stay alive and help a family during a devastating and impossible time. Matthew hasn't been the only child to wish to spend some time together with me, but he was the first and will always have a special place in my heart.

Thank you Matthew.

Another Dream Comes True: Barry Manilow

The first and only concert I ever attended as a child was to see Barry Manilow. My parents bought tickets for the family as a gift. At the time, my brother Larry's favorite artist was Ozzy Osbourne, so needless to say he wasn't as excited as I was. Our seats were very high up, only three rows from the back wall, but I was ecstatic. I loved Barry's songs and thought that his music was great. I aspired to be as good as Barry when I got older. As I watched the concert, I dreamed of being on stage and singing with him someday. Every child dreams of becoming like their heroes.

When I was younger I used to practice by vocalizing loudly to his songs in my room. During my illness my choir teacher, who also loved Barry's music, came to visit me in the hospital. He and I had our disagreements in the past, especially because he didn't believe that I was as sick as I was and had such a difficult time performing in his class. But our mutual respect and love for Manilow songs always gave us a common ground. We both appreciated the artistry and entertainment value of his work. When he walked into my hospital room, he handed me the newest Manilow cassette and that night I listened to a song called *Please Don't Be Scared*, which literally touched my soul. It was exactly what I needed to hear on that specific night. I felt like it was written just for me.

I had been fighting fear and depression for weeks and that song seemed to speak perfectly to my heart. I found myself listening to it often after that night and I credit it to being another piece of the puzzle of what saved my life during that time. Whenever I wanted to give up so the pain would stop, I would turn to music. In this instance it was Barry Manilow.

Years later, after my third single went to number one, I had the opportunity to sing that same song with Barry Manilow on a TV special he was shooting in Nashville. It hit me that night that my life was full of incredible moments that are almost impossible to explain or believe. I was transported back to that night when I was at the top row of his concert.

I wouldn't wish my illness on anyone, but I can honestly say that situations like these make life worth living, and without the fight, I may have never understood the true meaning of the value of enjoying every moment. There is great power in visualizing a dream in your mind until the day it actually happens. I fully realize that life is a precious gift that should be treasured every minute.

The Good The Bad and The Ugly

One of the greatest blessings in my life is the fact that every day I am able to be part of something that I love to do and am passionate about. However, that doesn't mean that it is not hard work, sometimes unfair and sometimes just plain ugly.

The thousands of kind words about my music, my performances or my courage have kept me afloat during the most difficult or emotionally draining times. I could be dragging along feeling like I can't go another step when a fan or someone who is in my corner will say the perfect words to breathe new energy into my day. There are so many times when I see someone standing in a line to get my autograph or to buy a concert ticket and I am overwhelmed with gratitude. If it were possible for me to thank every person individually I would.

One of the greatest and strangest compliments from a fan came from a young girl who had her orthodontist put my name and picture on her retainer! Other fans had outrageous requests for me, like signing body parts and much more. I must say the request was tempting, but I never really felt comfortable with that, so I didn't. It would have been easy for me to take advantage of many offers made to me by female fans and many times it was very tempting to my human nature, but for various reasons personal, professional and spiritual, I did not.

I remember the day I walked into the rehearsals for the American Music Awards, Dick Clark greeted me and said, "Kevin, I'm glad you're here!" I couldn't believe that Dick Clark knew my name. I could have died a happy man at that moment. I didn't get to see much of it because my seat was directly behind Shaquille O'Neal, but just having a reason to be in the same room with Shaq and so many other stars was exciting.

I was also nominated for an ACM award and a few other awards that year. I didn't win any of them, but my radio single, "Nobody Knows," was the most-played country song on radio and it won the BMI song of the year. That honor made up for the agony of defeat in the other categories. I was having too much fun to feel sorry for myself about a few awards. But I will say that it felt like being up for a great job promotion in front of all of your co-workers and then your boss telling you that you didn't get it. It does hurt some, particularly when millions of viewers know you didn't get it. However, I was doing concerts for thousands of fans that knew the lyrics to my songs by heart. I was singing duets and on stage with musical greats like Barry Manilow, Barbara Striesand, Celine Dion, Richard Marx and Josh Groban and I was writing songs with some of the worlds best writers. I was on top of the world.

As my career was on the rise so were exciting events. I was invited to be a guest on Regis and Kathy Lee. I was so excited because I was positive that Kathy Lee would truly "get me." I felt sure she would understand my struggle and excitement of reaching my dreams and the show would be fun. However, in true Kevin Sharp style, the day I was scheduled to be on the show, Regis had a substitute co-host; Joan Rivers. She didn't get me even a little bit, and admittedly, I didn't get her either, but I still had fun and felt privileged to be there. Maybe next time Kelly Rippa will be there to "get me!"

I was asked to be among the entertainers for one of Hollywood's "A" list parties. It was the 25th wedding anniversary of a movie studio bigwig. The performers were Faith Hill, Brandy, Michael Crawford and I. The guest list was something out of a dream - Tom Cruise, Nicole Kidman and Jim Carey to name a few. I was a nervous wreck. After my performance, all of the "beautiful people" complimented me and thanked me for being there. Then a really amazing thing happened. I needed to be back in New York for another show the following day, so the nice folks at Time Warner lent me the corporate jet to get me there in time. Michael Crawford asked me if he could hitch a ride to Las Vegas on the way. (I graciously agreed to let him share my jet.) It was incredible. A personal chef prepared a great meal and the flight attendant showed me to my room where I slept until we reached New York. I felt like Elvis getting off that plane, even though I could see the disappointment in the faces of the people anxiously awaiting the arrival of a mega star. They were looking at each other saying, "Who is that?" I knew then that I was definitely in New York! It was evident that I had more work to do in the publicity arena. Even so, it was the greatest flight of my life and it made it hard to go back to commercial flights after that!

Duty Calls

Recently, I was asked to sing for the President of the United States (George W. Bush) and thirty thousand military troops. When I said yes, I was told that the performance was the next day. I didn't realize that the President's whereabouts are not common knowledge, and everything is done on the QT. The next day, I found myself traveling from Cincinnati, Ohio to Fort Polk, Louisiana. The government did a background check on me using my social security number and birth certificate. I didn't think I had a shady background, but if I did, they seemed the type of men who would find it, and I was about to find out!

John Berry was also asked to perform. As it turns out, both John and I had family members stationed at that base to help make our appearances possible, so it was really special for both of us. When we arrived at the base we were met by very professional military personnel who escorted us to our destination, briefed us on protocol while in the company of the President, and passed us through metal detectors. It was very unnerving. Then we waited for hours until it was time to sing. Imagine how long it takes for thirty thousand soldiers to go through metal detectors! It's not a quick process.

I had performed in front of thousands of people many times before, but this was different. Seeing that many people in military uniforms awaiting their opportunity to see the Commander in Chief, not to mention the many snipers on the rooftops of each building, was awe-inspiring. Even though I was fully aware that the snipers were there for the safety of the President, and there was probably no safer place on the planet at that moment, I still felt uneasy. Because I was nervous, I said a few things that I thought would be funny, like "I hate the Marines," but soon found out that the Armed Forces don't have rivalries with other branches like college football teams.

They weren't amused.   Oops, now I know.

After I sang, I couldn't tell if they liked me or not, but I could tell that I felt a sense of pride and gratitude for every person serving our country.   I will never forget that feeling of overwhelming appreciation for the troops.   After the President began his speech, he stopped to thank John and me for our performances.   I was once again, overwhelmed and filled with joy.

Because John and I had a background check, we were able to meet the President. Our guests were not allowed to come with us and we were not permitted to bring our cameras either.   We were reminded not to make any sudden movements and to move down the reception line quickly. After he took pictures with a few military and government officials, it was finally our turn to say hello.   I was silently practicing being brief.   Then he took pictures with me and continued to talk to me for seven minutes!!   I was shocked.   He asked about my health, told me he was a big country music fan, and we talked about my career. I was very impressed with him as being a kind and wonderful man regardless of politics and world events. I was so nervous I couldn't remember half of the details of our conversation.

As we were about to leave, I asked a secret service man if I could give him my address to send me a copy of a picture of me and the President. He just looked at me and said, "Don't worry Mr. Sharp, we know where you live." I think he was trying to freak me out. A few months later a picture arrived in the mail. I guess secret service men don't lie!

Would You Like Fries With That?

There is no doubt that being in my position as a country music artist has given me opportunities for exciting and excellent experiences. I cherish every good time, compliment, and pat on the back. However, it also opens up my life to many people who aren't so nice or those who feel it is their responsibility to point out my faults and weaknesses.

I have run into fans from all walks of life and most of them are wonderful and I am blessed to meet them, however, sometimes there is a character that makes me suspect that I am on a hidden camera reality show. For example, this one time after a long drive home from a visit with my wife Traci's family, I was at a fast food restaurant drive-thru and the girl at the window told me I looked like Kevin Sharp. I didn't know what to say besides, "I am Kevin Sharp," but without missing a beat she said, "No you're not. He's not that chubby." I was in a state of shock, so I replied, "He is now."

Meanwhile, Traci was snickering in the seat next to me, and if that wasn't bad enough, the girl says to me, "I am one of Kevin's biggest fans. His teeth aren't as crooked as yours and he has blue eyes."

Now Traci was doubled over with laughter, calling her Mom on her cell phone to tell her what was happening. At this point I was so frustrated, I pulled out my wallet to show her my driver's license to which she replied, "You had that made." I could not believe that she would suspect someone of going to the DMV to stand in line to get a fake Kevin Sharp license. By this time, Tracy was laughing so hard she could hardly breathe. I was so caught off guard by this gal's insistence that I was trying to dupe her, that I took a CD and picture from the back of my car and autographed it and gave it to her. I was sure this would prove my identity and she would finally believe me. I was ready to calm her embarrassment by being very friendly to her. This was not the case. As we were pulling away from the window, she yelled, "If you were really Kevin Sharp, you would be driving a nicer car."

By the time I left that window I was so beat up and felt two inches tall. A "fan" had attacked my appearance, my character and worst of all, my Lincoln LS, which until that day, I was very happy with. Traci howled with laughter all the way home. Ain't fame great?

Lemonade

Everyone knows the adage, "When life hands you lemons - make lemonade," and for the most part, I believe that the theory behind it is a great message. It is very important to walk through life with a positive outlook using one's ability to make the best of a bad situation.

However, I have to admit that there was a time when I thought I would drown if I had to swallow any more lemonade. In fact, I could write a recipe book when it comes to lemons! Sometimes I have been bombarded by them from every side. My ability to see the humor, blessing, or lesson in some of my "situations" admittedly has eluded me.

Sometimes I have felt and still feel down right angry - angry at the world, angry at God, angry at my family, angry with my doctors, and many times, angry with myself. I am enraged at the fact that there are no answers to unfair and mind-boggling circumstances.

Why do bad things happen to good people? Why do families have to suffer the loss of a child? How can we discover so many things through science and technology, but still have no ability to save a child from an illness or accident?

All of these questions plague me. However, I have come to the conclusion that if I need to find answers or have a desire to help in some small way, I must first accept the fact that sometimes there just are no reasons, and life just happens.

I was under the impression from a young age that if I was a good, moral and upstanding person striving to achieve what is right; I would never come face to face with disaster. I was wrong. No one is exempt from the trials in life. Some trials are big and some are small, but there will always be trials.

Cancer hit me like a ton of bricks. Losing Kelley and Matthew and so many others affected me in ways that no words on paper could ever describe.

But, I press on, and no, that does not mean I make lemonade. I have learned to juggle! Sometimes I find myself having to juggle several lemons at one time. Many times I drop them and just sit among them and cry.

I have chosen to wake up every morning seeking a chance to lend a word of kindness or encouragement to someone in a bad situation. I don't do it out of some noble gesture toward mankind. I do it out of a desire to keep my sanity. Most of my opportunities have been with people fighting or surviving cancer and I am grateful for that. I try to administer a little hope along the way and usually find a lot of hope in return. It is the hope that allows me to keep juggling.

Most cancer survivors share a common bond not only in "war stories," but also in after-effects of chemo and in the reality of chronic pain.   My leg has been in pain since before I was ever diagnosed and to my recollection the pain has never gone away.   The cancer is gone, but the pain remains. My radiation treatments had not only killed the cancer, but also the surrounding tissue. My pain is permanent. Those lemons wait for me at the foot of my bed every morning, and follow me around all day, every day.

For those who have never dealt with chronic pain for at least a year, there is no way to explain the shadow it casts on every day life.   Living with pain becomes a lifestyle.   Daily events are planned around doses of medicine, the distance from one place to the next, and a body position that will cause the least amount of discomfort while sleeping in bed; are crucial considerations.

After a while if I let my guard down, I could suffer from depression and despair. I have that right. After all, I am carrying a bushel of lemons around with me all day.

I choose not to. I have been down the depression road and it was ugly and much more difficult to travel that anyone can imagine.

I was fortunate enough, with the help of understanding family and friends, to come through it. Going back is not an option for me.

Instead, I am constantly seeking ways to use my familiarity in the public eye as a tool to help those who, like me, need support. I am blessed to be able to record my songs and to have a chance to make my mark in the music industry. I never take that for granted or assume in any way that I did anything to deserve the recognition. That is why I never use the word "famous" to describe what I am or ever want to be. Famous conjures up thoughts of being some untouchable, self-absorbed icon that keeps everyone at arm's length. That is not who I am. I strive solely to be familiar. Someone who is approachable and friendly, that wants to know people, not waiting for my ovation, but wanting to applaud those who press on through tough times. I want a person to recognize me as someone who cares deeply about the well-being of others and who wishes to help. I am no different from anyone else who makes it through the day that is fraught with twists and turns. I just happen to be a familiar singer that can juggle lemons!

A Ray of Light

We all know the expression, "The light at the end of the tunnel." I know I have spent a large amount of my life praying that pain would stop or that fog and darkness would lift. I have struggled with many trials and sometimes found it hard to see even a tiny crack of light break the pitch black.

Many times I questioned myself as to whether there really was a light or if I would recognize it if I stumbled upon it. I have gone weeks upon weeks doubting that I could survive, hating my very existence, and feeling sorry for myself. I have spent many days unwilling to pray because I didn't believe that it would change anything. However, through all of my depressions and fears and loathing's, there was always one thing that flickered ever so lightly in the back of my mind and depths of my heart and that was "hope." Sometimes it was no more than a dying ember, which was sometimes dangerously close to burning out, but it was there.

Many times my fear or anger had nothing to do with my personal circumstances. I would walk through the hospital Pediatrics Ward and not understand why those kids were there. I pondered the accidental death of a dear friend and felt so angry and helpless. I didn't understand why things like suicide, drug overdoses, suffering, murder or even war exist. I know that there are people in the world that wrestle with the thought of getting out of bed in the morning, whose every thought is a fight to make it through another day in chronic pain or sadness. I am positive about one thing - hope is the gift that God has given us to make it to tomorrow. It is the one thing that humans have that can crack the sky and let a ray of light in and overcome a dark situation. As long as hope is alive, even the worst situation can be overcome.

I have learned more about myself during the writing of this book than I have in all the years of actually living. By remembering long forgotten details, and allowing old feelings to resurface, I have put many things to rest and forgiven God and myself for so many "unfair" dealings. I have a truer understanding of what is important.

I have realized that people in general are more alike than they are different. It is usually the media or society that tries to tell us who we should love and who we should hate, but that is not reality. These decisions should be self-founded and personal. If we really got to know each other it would be very difficult to hate at all. We can see a little bit of ourselves in everyone out there if we take the time to look. We all hurt, we all love, and we all have to deal with life's "surprises." None of us are superior because of the job we do, the money we have or the lifestyle we live. God is not concerned with status, physical beauty or fame. To Him we are all the same. We are all subject to trials and thankfully we are all equally as subject to His love and kindness. Hope and prayer are two tools that God gives to everyone. It is our willingness to use them or not use them that separates us or joins us together.

I hope you have been able to see a part of yourself in this book. I hope you recognize your own troubles and triumphs through the situations I have endured. I ask you to forgive yourself of the 100 mistakes you might make today and strive to make only 99 tomorrow. Forgive those too.

Please know that you are loved more than you can imagine, and that when you are at your lowest and weakest point. that is when hope will change everything. Tragedy can truly bring the greatest gifts into our lives if we are willing to see them.

Thank you for taking time in your life to spend a little time in mine. Remember to love those around you and never be afraid to dream great things for your future. Remember, "You have something left to do."

May God bless you and yours.

Kevin

Survival Equation

If it isn't already obvious by now, you should know that I don't have all the answers or some secret formula to share with you. I don't have a simple solution that explains why I'm still here when so many others have lost their lives to cancer. Although I will tell you what I believe made the difference for me.

When I sit down and add it all up, I find that medical science and technology was a small part of the equation. I believe that it wasn't so much the medications I was being given as it was how and who was giving them to me. So many times it was the comforting words from a doctor, a nurse or just an employee of the hospital that made the difference. It was the silence of the nurse who decided to read a book by my bedside on her/his lunch break. It was the many friends who spent hours with me, thinking only of me in place of the other things and responsibilities they had in their lives.

It goes without saying that I needed my family camping out at my bedside at different times. I needed my father, who spent three weeks straight without leaving my side early in my diagnosis. I would love to give personal credit to each and every family member, every friend and caregiver who played a roll in my survival. However, it would double the length of this book and more importantly, I fear I would leave someone out. You know who you are and I thank you from the bottom of my heart.

When it's all said and done, it was the simple things and acts of love that gave me the strength to fight and press on into my battle, with my whole heart and soul. For those who need a visual equation I believe this is what it would look like.

SOME + <u>FAMILY</u> X <u>LOVE</u> = HOPE & MEDICAL FRIENDS FAITH SURVIVAL SCIENCE